FIGHTING WEIGHT

FIGHTING WEIGHT

How I Achieved Healthy Weight Loss with "Banding," a New Procedure That Eliminates Hunger—Forever

Khaliah Ali

Dr. George Fielding, Dr. Christine Ren,
Lawrence Lindner

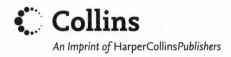

An Imprint of HarperCollins*Publishers*

"Reunited" by Frederick J. Perren and Dino Fekaris © 1978 Bibo Music Publishing, Inc. and Perren-Vibes Music, Inc. All rights administered by Universal-Polygram International Publishing, Inc./ ASCAP Used By Permission. All Right Reserved; Ford Model Photograph of Khaliah Ali, Courtesy of Ford Models, Inc.; Khaliah Ali with her father and Lou Schwartz, Courtesy of the American Sportscasters Association; Photograph of Khaliah Ali with Don King, Ted Turner, Roy Innis, Marcia Clark, and Robert Merrill, Courtesy of the Congress of Racial Equality/Tom Casino; Illustrations (3) of an open surgery incision, of laparascopic incisions, and of the gastric band placed near top of stomach, Courtesy of Allergan Medical; Cover of the *Simplicity* catalog, Courtesy of Simplicity Patterns Company, Inc., Photograph of Khaliah Ali with Kenneth Cole, Courtesy of Randy Brooke/ WireImage.com; Photograph of Khaliah Ali at an event for the National Center for Missing and Exploited Children, Courtesy of the National Center for Missing and Exploited Children; Photograph of Khaliah Ali with Dionne Warwick, ©PatrickMcMullan.com; Photograph of Khaliah Ali with "Peacemaker" bike, LynnJonesFoundation.org.

HarperCollins books may be purchased for educational, business, or sales promotional use. For information, please write: Special Markets Department, HarperCollins Publishers, 10 East 53rd Street, New York, NY 10022.

FIRST EDITION

Designed by Jaime Putorti

Library of Congress Cataloging-in-Publication Data

Ali, Khaliah.
    Fighting weight : how I achieved healthy weight loss with "banding," a new procedure that eliminates hunger—forever / Khaliah Ali, Christine Ren and George Felding ; with Lawrence Lindner.
        p. cm.
    ISBN: 978-0-06-117094-2
    ISBN-10: 0-06-117094-1
    1. Ali, Khaliah—Health. 2. Overweight women—United States—Biography. 3. Jejunoileal bypass—Patients—United States—Biography. I. Ren, Christine. II. Fielding, George. III. Title.

RC628.A43 2007
362.196'3980092—dc22
[B]

2007060870

To my son, Jacob—
And to all children whose parents have opted out
of too many photos with them

CONTENTS

FIGHTING WEIGHT

CLAIMING YOUR LIFE

Twenty million Americans can't pull an airplane seat belt across their laps. They can't run for a train, can't step into the bathtub without great deliberation, and can't push a child on a swing. Nor can they sit on a bistro chair or other fragile furniture because, quite simply, they'd break it. Most don't dare go to the beach, wear sleeveless shirts, hold out hope for true romance, or enjoy being in public.

All are candidates for weight-loss surgery. Beside the everyday mortification of literally not being able to fit into life, they're susceptible to heart disease, diabetes, arthritis, interruptions in breathing during sleep, and a host of other debilitating, if not life-threatening, conditions.

Still, less than 1 percent of those eligible for obesity surgery come forward, largely because they fear the risks of the operation. I was one of them.

I know firsthand the shame of becoming morbidly obese; the lifetime of dieting off pounds, but never enough, and then gaining them all back and more; the aching joints, the inability to walk up a single flight of stairs without losing my breath—all made worse by the fact that I was the daughter of a man who is very famous, in large part, precisely because of his fitness and physical abilities. I remember well, too, the experience of finally coming around to the idea of weight-loss surgery but rejecting it because of the very real possibility that I would die on the table.

A year after I gave birth to my son, Jacob, I ballooned up to my highest weight ever—325 pounds. I feared for my life. I feared for my son, worrying that he would grow up without his mother. I feared going on any more diets because, as I learned all too well, very, very few people can diet off more than 100 pounds—and keep them off. And I feared gastric bypass surgery because one in two hundred patients doesn't recover from it, a risk that was just too great.

Frightened and miserable, I went five years losing and gaining the same fifty pounds and didn't know which way to turn—until a wonderful friend steered me toward Drs. George Fielding and Christine Ren, professors at the New York University School of Medicine. My friend told me they performed a type of weight-loss surgery that has been used in Europe for more than a decade but is only now starting to take off in the United States. The results of the surgery are just as spectacular as those of gastric bypass, she said, yet with only one-tenth the rate of life-threatening complications.

I didn't believe her. But desperate, I did finally read about Drs. Fielding and Ren on the Internet. Then I went to see them, propelled in part by the fact that they have performed more of this European type of weight-loss procedure than any other doctors in the world. (More recently, their practice was named one of only four "better performers" out of twenty-nine bariatric surgery practices rated by the very prestigious University Healthcare Consortium.)

Soon, with their record of success and also their hand-holding through my own hand-wringing, they convinced me of the procedure's safety, and I was on the road to slimming down to a goal weight of 150 pounds—not bad for a woman who's five feet nine inches.

I have a debt of gratitude to Drs. Fielding and Ren that can never be repaid. How can you repay someone for giving you your life? So, when they asked me to do this book with them as a way of dramatizing what a very obese person goes through—and how she can come out "the other side"—I was thrilled to take part. Please be aware as you read that while the story is mine, all the scientific facts, figures, research, and medical explanations are theirs.

THE EUROPEAN SOLUTION TO OBESITY

The type of procedure I underwent is called laparoscopic adjustable gastric banding, or gastric banding, for short. (You can also call it stomach banding, because that's what it is.) It doesn't involve stapling your stomach and cutting your intestine in two, as does gastric bypass—the surgery chosen by such notables as Carnie Wilson and Al Roker. Instead, it's relatively low-tech as operations go. A band is simply placed around the stomach and periodically tightened to reduce hunger sensations, as well as limit the amount of food you can process at one time. That's it.

The operation was perfected by Dr. Fielding, who *developed* the technique that is presently used worldwide to implant the band. It offers myriad advantages over gastric bypass.

1. **It's reversible.** If you don't like the band, you can have it removed. Gastric bypass, by contrast, is a decision you usually can't go back on because the complication rate for reversing the surgery is too risky.

2. Low rate of postoperative problems. There are fewer adverse effects from the operation and even fewer deaths— one in two thousand, as opposed to gastric bypass's one in two hundred.

3. More patient follow-up because you need to have the band tightened every so often. It's a simple outpatient procedure that involves no anesthesia, just an injection of watery solution that thickens the band so it can wrap a little tighter around the stomach. I've had mine tightened a number of times now. It's about as eventful as getting your teeth cleaned.

4. No hunger. With gastric bypass, hunger eventually returns because the stomach softens up, or "stretches," and there's nothing that can be done, which is why the weight of most people who have gastric bypass drifts upward again. With gastric banding, the periodic band tightening keeps hunger at bay *forever* so the weight can keep coming off as you need, and *stay* off. Even dieting plateaus don't sabotage the weight-loss effort. Usually, when obese people reach a plateau and stop losing weight for a while, the hunger combined with the disappointment of not seeing the scale needle move downward decreases motivation, so weight starts to creep back up. I know the pattern all too well. But with the band, the plateau is bearable. It can be waited out until the next drop in pounds because there's no hunger involved.

5. No dumping. With gastric bypass, eating even a tiny amount of a sugary food, less than a single bite's worth, can cause dumping—a precipitous drop in blood sugar that results in the sweats, nausea, and often a very scary feeling of panic.

I know people who have gone through it. It doesn't happen after banding surgery.

6. No nutritional deficiencies. With gastric bypass, you have to take vitamin and mineral supplements for the rest of your life because the surgery creates permanent nutrient malabsorption. With gastric banding, a simple multivitamin that millions of Americans already take is recommended to provide nutritional "insurance."

7. Safer pregnancy. For pregnancy as well as breast-feeding, the band can simply be loosened to allow for the right intake of calories and nutrients. It's that simple—and also makes it easier for many once-obese women to *become* pregnant, since excess weight often keeps them from conceiving in the first place. The pregnancy itself goes much more smoothly, too. In a study out of the Australian Center for Obesity Research and Education in Melbourne, 42 percent of women carrying a child prior to getting a stomach band had pregnancy-induced hypertension, and 11 percent ended up with gestational diabetes. During pregnancies after band surgery, only 11 percent suffered pregnancy-induced hypertension and only 6 percent developed gestational diabetes. What's more, after the band surgeries there were fewer stillbirths, abnormal-weight babies, and other complications.

Other benefits of gastric banding surgery: the operation takes an hour or less, whereas gastric bypass requires two to three hours under anesthesia. Furthermore, you're out of the hospital in one day (as opposed to two to three days) and back at work within a week. I was on the *Today* show talking with Ann Curry, Dr. Fielding by my side, just four days after my own procedure. With gastric bypass, it could be up to three weeks before you're able to resume your normal activities.

The recovery goes so fast because the operation does not entail rearranging your internal organs, the way gastric bypass does. As Dr. Ren says, the band simply acts as an effective appetite suppressant without the side effects of appetite-suppressing drugs. "This is not a grandstanding operation," she explains. "It's a very gentle procedure, a facilitator to diet and exercise rather than a body punisher."

She personally loves doing it because while training as a surgeon, she saw people come into the office so happy after obesity surgery. "They would hug you," she says. "You don't see this in surgeons' offices. Most of the surgery you see right now is cancer surgery. *This* operation, by contrast, is not lifesaving but life-*giving*. I wanted to be in on that—that happiness, the confidence, the amazing transformations people experience. They exude confidence and happiness that they didn't have before. They *stand* taller."

Currently, only one out of five weight-loss operations in the United States is a gastric banding, as opposed to four out of five in Europe. Why? One reason is that gastric banding has been standard in Europe since the mid-1990s (and is also easily available in Australia and other countries) but was approved here only in 2001. But beyond that, surgeons do the surgeries they know. While Americans were perfecting the gastric bypass (an operation first performed in the 1960s, after doctors observed that removing part of the stomach as a cancer treatment or ulcer therapy led to weight loss), doctors in other countries were cultivating the gastric band.

THE EASY WAY OUT?

A lot of people believe opting for obesity surgery is taking the easy way out, just one more sign that very fat people lack willpower. Again, I was one of them.

Like both fat and thin people everywhere, I had bought into the idea that thin people have more self-control than heavy ones, that they're more together. In other words, I believed I simply wasn't trying hard enough, couldn't stick with anything, and was living a sloppy, unstructured life and therefore deserved to remain miserable, constantly out of breath, my knees and feet always in pain, and being the subject of people's cruel stares and even crueler comments.

That belief, in fact, was part of the reason I hesitated before undergoing the operation that finally helped me lose the weight I needed to lose. It was subtler than the fear but still insistent, and kept wearing me down and making it impossible for me to act. I was convinced that to lose weight by surgery instead of diet and exercise would be "cheating," in short, proof that I hadn't *really* taken hold of my life and was instead "surrendering" to my lesser self.

I was wrong. I *was* trying hard enough—my entire life. From the time I was five years old and a friend told me I wouldn't be so "blubbery" if I didn't eat so much blubbery steak, I dieted. I was even trotted out in front of Jane Pauley on the *Today* show as a nine-year-old as part of a program to slim down overweight kids.

As an adult, I dieted on my own, at one point taking off almost a hundred pounds. But the weight always came back.

Dr. Fielding had gone through the same thing. Fat from childhood, he lost—and gained—seventy pounds *four times* as an adult before opting for the very gastric banding surgery he had already performed on hundreds of others.

Our experience is often true of obese people. They spend more energy on dieting, *starving,* working to control hunger, than anyone else. And most of them do lose thirty, forty, fifty pounds—many times over—exhibiting a lot more willpower than most thin people have ever had to show.

So what do thin people have over those who are extremely overweight, if not self-control? Luck. Or, more specifically, genetic luck. The genes that put their ancestors at grave health risk thousands of years ago, by making it difficult to hold on to fat stores in times of food scarcity, are the very genes that are keeping them thin and largely free of health risks today in the face of food overabundance.

Thin and even mildly overweight people often scoff at that notion, as I know all too well. They say that while a person's genes could perhaps cause a weight gain of twenty, thirty, or even fifty pounds, there's no way someone's genetics could cause her to gain a hundred or more excess pounds. The fault for such obesity, they say, falls on the eater's lack of resolve, not her own particular metabolic circumstances. Not true, and you need only to look at the growing ranks of the obese over the last seventy years to douse such thinking.

As Dr. Fielding likes to tell it, if you had said to your thin, tough grandparents in 1935 that they would be able to sit in their car, make the window go down with a flick of a finger rather than with a hand crank, and have a nice teenager hand all their grandchildren five thousand calories through the window with none of them making a single move, they'd have told you to stop dreaming. That is, seventy years ago, constant availability of very high-calorie food with no need to expend any calories in order to procure that food was inconceivable, and there were extremely few obese people.

What has changed in the last several decades is not people's level of willpower but our food supply, which has literally become toxic. It's now nothing, as I know intimately, to buy an 1,100-calorie pecan bun from Cinnabon's, an 850-calorie Taco Bell taco salad, a 600-calorie king-size fries, a 400-calorie slice of pizza topped with pepperoni, or a 1,200-calorie pint of superrich ice cream. And there are no more scheduled mealtimes around the table to cue you about when eating starts and when it's over. It's all grazing, all the time. Furthermore, it is more common now to overeat for emotional reasons.

It's at the intersection of these changes that the genetic differences come in. Some people can eat whatever they want whenever they want with no consequences on the scale, or at least not severe consequences. Their metabolic wiring allows them to burn calories faster. Or they may have hormones that are set in such a way that they simply do not get as hungry as other people or as turned on by the sight of food. Others, like me, are not so fortunate. And the not-so-fortunate number keeps growing, because as the food supply keeps getting more and more abundant and concentrated in calories (not to mention more available at every turn), more and more people's genes and metabolisms are losing the ability to withstand the caloric onslaught. Their internal signals are overridden.

In 1980, 15 percent of Americans were obese; now it's more than 30 percent. What has changed is the food, along with the drop in the number of calories people burn in daily activities—not their characters, genes, willpower, or anything else.

How bad can it get? Ninety percent of human beings have the potential to become obese or morbidly obese. Only about 10 percent are resistant to all the extra calories available. Those lucky 10 percent fit into one of two analogies. Either they're like Toyotas in a gasoline crisis, getting by perfectly fine on less, while the rest of us are like SUVs, guzzling fuel (that happens to be much cheaper than the fuel for our vehicles, a lethal bargain). *Or* they have SUV appetites but burn their food calories so fast they have Toyota figures.

Okay, you might say, some people, maybe even most people, are more vulnerable to becoming very overweight. But why can't obese people diet off the excess pounds? (Or, as I've heard expressed behind my back in audible, disgusted stage whispers, "She could at least lose fifty pounds.") The answer is not clear-cut and not yet well understood. But the research community is making inroads. One thing that seems apparent is that the threshold for hunger resets once someone becomes very overweight, so the body needs more food more frequently to feel sated. It could also be that the gastrointestinal tract becomes less sensitive to hormones that regulate appetite. Perhaps there's some other biological explanation that's waiting to be discovered. In the meantime, what's known for certain is that while someone who is moderately overweight can successfully shed twenty, thirty, even sometimes forty or fifty pounds, chasing away seventy, eighty, a hundred or more pounds—and keeping them off—is virtually impossible.

That's not to say it never happens. It does. But the success stories are phenomenally rare, much more rare than even many in the medical community are willing to admit. Those photos on magazines at the supermarket checkout of people who have shed a hundred pounds—it's a statistical fact that only 2 percent of them are able to keep off the weight. And the constant hunger and deprivation those successful 2 percent must put themselves through are often more than anyone should have to bear. It's like living with another kind of eating disorder. Those photos actually do a great disservice, because they only fuel the false notion that if obese people just tried hard enough, they could take off the weight. I know they used to get me down—after the initial, short-lived spiral into "hopeful."

Whatever weight I lost always came back, whatever effort I put into it always backfired. Even the most extraordinary effort was no match for the tenacity of my obese body. The hunger my body engendered was like the subject in Edvard Munch's painting *The Scream*. It was constant; it was maddening; it always got the better of me.

DAMNED ONLY IF YOU DON'T

I suffered countless indignities because of society's accusing finger, compounding the physical and emotional misery my weight caused—

poor treatment and withering stares from salespeople, askance looks from physicians in examining rooms, a smug unwillingness of people to hold open an elevator door, all adding to the severe depression and social isolation. When I finally did opt for surgery, a lot of people blamed me once again, for going the route of a quick fix rather than doing the hard work. It was like I was trying to get out of my "punishment." I was damned for not being able to lose weight without medical intervention and then damned again for availing myself of the tool that allowed me to achieve what the entire world said I should have been achieving my whole life. But even the National Institutes of Health have gone on record saying that for morbidly obese people, surgery is the only hope. The American College of Surgeons and other health-promoting organizations support obesity surgery, too. Medicare, the health insurance program for older people, now pays for it (and private health insurers often follow Medicare's lead, which means there's a good chance that more and more health insurance companies will begin to reimburse for the procedure).

Besides, it's not a quick fix. After obesity surgery, you still have to eat healthfully. You still have to exercise. You still have to pay attention to your body's signals every single day. The difference is that **the surgery creates a level playing field. It finally gives very large people the tool that everyone else takes for granted—the ability to not feel hungry every minute of every day** so that they can once and for all get their eating under control.

In other words, if you do choose gastric banding, you're not ducking responsibility. You're not surrendering, and you're not weak. You're finally *taking charge* by making use of a device that can help you. You're claiming the life that everybody else kept telling you how to live.

That's what I want to talk to you about—claiming, or enrolling in, your own life. Think about the fruitless battles you can do with your body over years, over *decades,* then making a choice for *allowing* your body to cooperate with you so that all your thwarted dreams can become your reality. That's a choice I finally made, not in surrender and weakness but in fierce, levelheaded determination, and it has not damned me. It *sustains* me. I've never been happier than I am now.

It goes way beyond the frivolous things, like being able to wear whatever I want, although I take great pleasure in details like that. But what I also love is being able to walk into a room and not get snickered at. I love having the energy to play catch with my son, to take him trick-or-treating on Halloween and not feel self-conscious, to present a business idea to a team of investors without feeling that my weight is more convincing of the idea's failure than my words of its success. I love getting to live many years more than I might very well have been destined to live as a morbidly obese person. Most of all, I love being at peace with myself.

As for any person who has dealt with obesity, it was not an easy journey. And being a daughter of one of the world's most famous and admired people didn't shield me. In fact, in certain ways it only put me more in the spotlight, perhaps in more negative ways than other people of size. From the time I was in grade school, I was taunted by peers, even hit by other kids, because I was "big" and therefore could "fight like my father."

Nothing could have been further from the truth. I hung back, partly because I was a gentle kid but also because I wouldn't have been able to bear drawing that kind of attention to myself. Not now. I *like* being with other people, whether it's hanging out with friends, conducting business, or making a speech to raise money for a charitable organization. And I like being romantically available, as well as available to participate in physical activities, which had always been closed to me before. That is, I like where my journey has taken me, and continues to take me.

I realize it's not the same for all large people, and that not all of them are even intent on losing weight. Some, while they may at one or more points in their lives have tried to slim down, have joined what is commonly called the Size Acceptance Movement. Despite the profound bigotry against them (it is still acceptable to loathe fat people openly, to make fun of them, to deny them jobs and promotions), despite all the health risks, they are able to make peace with their bodies and de-emphasize the role of eating and weight in their lives. They find a way to move forward even while dealing with the physical and societal limitations. To them, I—and Drs. Fielding and Ren—say, "Our best to you." No one should ever be pushed into doing anything she or he doesn't want to.

But most very large people are very unhappy about their bodies, their health, their looks, the prejudice against them. They would do anything if only they could lose the weight. They think about it every waking moment. That's who I'm talking to in this book. And I, who previously had not even been able to experience physical intimacy without artfully draping myself so as to be more or less hidden from view at those very moments when a person is supposed to feel free and unfettered, am here to tell you that you don't have to live that way. You can change the course of your journey, too.

I know, because my story is your story. While the details may be different, you'll recognize the arc of despair. You'll see, however, that you can rewrite all the chapters yet to come.

1

"BLUBBERY"

Reunited and it feels so good
Reunited 'cause we understood
There's one perfect fit
And, sugar, this one is it . . .

Peaches & Herb's number-one hit was wafting over from the radio on the kitchen windowsill. I had just turned five, the trees had all leafed out for early summer, and I was sitting with my best friend, Teddy, on the deck behind the house on Philadelphia's Main Line that my father had bought for my mother and me not long before.

It was one of those perfect childhood moments that you can count on one hand. Both Teddy and I had fathers we didn't always get to be with (his was Teddy Pendergrass), but our mothers were very close, to the point that I often called his mom not simply my aunt but Mama Rose, and he called mine Mama Aaisha.

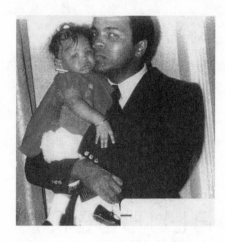

MY FIRST CHRISTMAS. THAT
DRESS WAS RED VELVET.

Many days we'd all pile into the car and go to the beach together, with Teddy and me nodding off on each other's shoulders during the ride back home from the Jersey shore and then being plopped onto a big bed. Some nights, one of our mothers would get a bushel of crabs, and we'd eat, dance to oldies, watch television, then sit up late and talk. For a year or so Teddy and I took the same school bus, and once he and his friends handcuffed me to a bench for a prank, with the bus company having to call the police to unhitch me. When we'd have sleepovers, I used to snore, and he would hold my lips shut until I couldn't breathe and would wake up. We truly loved and teased each other like brother and sister. My mother and I even lived at Teddy Pendergrass's home for several months one year when our pipes burst and the house flooded and then took forever to fix.

So when we were all together and our mothers were happy, as they were that summer day, I felt enveloped in that blissful note of security that only a child can feel wrapped in so warmly.

Our mothers had just finished barbecuing steaks on the grill. I was happily chewing my heart out, particularly because my own mother had recently given in to my grandmother and stopped trying to raise me on a strictly vegan diet, without any meat or dairy. This was one steak I didn't have to sneak on Grandmom's watch.

I especially loved the meat right by the gristle, where it tasted saltier and juicier. My soul was literally swaying to my eating, to the air that hadn't yet turned too humid, to the music . . .

As we reminisce
On precious moments like this
I'm glad we're back together—

"That's why you're so blubbery. Because you eat all that blubbery steak."

Teddy jolted me from my reverie, and from much else. It was the first time someone had so bluntly made me feel there was something unacceptable about me.

Suddenly I felt conscious of my bare arms poking through my favorite sleeveless sundress, the heat rising to my face. I put down my fork.

In truth, my weight as a topic wasn't entirely new to me. My mother had already begun to show concern.

Part of it was that were we built so differently. My mother, like her sister and all her cousins, had a lithe frame and was petite. But I was built big, like my father's side, and looked a lot like him and his mother, whom everyone called Mama Bird and who was quite heavy. In fact, the day I was born—Father's Day, 1974—my father took one look at me and said, "Oh my God, she's a Little Bird." It became my nickname as well as my legacy. Even by the time I was two or three, I was a chunkier child than others, and I was clearly chubby by the time I hit kindergarten.

It wasn't just my weight that alarmed my mother; it was my

height. I was *so* tall for my age, to the point that by the time I reached first grade, my feet were bigger than hers. I couldn't fit into her shoes, the way little girls like to do when playing pretend dress-up. And I think that fueled the "Oh my God, she's big" notion. My mother just didn't *understand* my body.

My weight and size were not the only things that concerned her. Although quite thin by the time I was born, she had been a very chubby child with Coke-bottle glasses, praised for her braininess but not her looks. All that changed, however, when she came down with rheumatic fever at age thirteen and was sick in bed for the better part of a year. She lost a lot of weight as a result of the disease, learned to compensate without her glasses, and literally emerged from the illness radiant. Overnight, so to speak, she turned into a swan that garnered a lot of attention for her looks. And having learned first-hand the value of attractiveness—it was much of what initially drew my father to her, after all—she feared my missing out on that asset, as she had earlier in life.

So she dieted me, as she was constantly dieting herself, eating tiny portions and exercising excessively. In fact, I feel pretty confi-

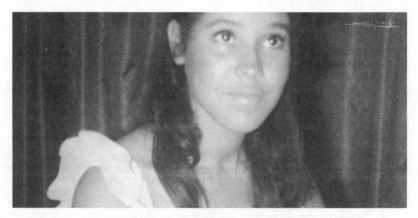

MY MOTHER NOT LONG AFTER SHE MET MY FATHER.

dent that my mother's vegan phase was, at least in part, an effort to control her weight.

She didn't actually put me on structured calorie-controlled plans, at least not early on, but she was always making an effort to limit the amount I ate. I remember lots of negotiating, coupled with lots of "getting caught."

"You can have two Girl Scout cookies."

"Okay, Mom."

Then she'd walk out of the room, and I'd take a handful— nothing will make you eat more than being told you can't. When she came back in, she'd say, predictably, "You ate these."

"No, I didn't."

"Yes, you did. I counted them. You're going to get fat."

Other times she'd withhold by taking inventory on how much food was left in a container or a package. "This orange juice had been nearly full. How much are you drinking?" Or, "How many slices of cheese did you take?" I was always scared she'd come up behind me and ask, "How much of this did you have?"

It made me feel like I was bad—and ugly. And the feeling of ugliness was only heightened by the fact that my mother was so incredibly beautiful. All kids think their moms are perfect—mystical, beautiful creatures. But mine really was otherworldly in her person— long, silky hair, very keen features, and smooth, perfect olive skin. At the same time, she was fresh-faced, the kind of woman who beguiled without a touch of makeup.

And there I was, doughy-faced, with chubby cheeks and pigtails. My hair was trainable, but not as luxurious, or as luxuriously long, as hers.

I think those feelings of inadequacy contributed greatly to my love of fashion today. It doesn't surprise me, looking back, that I ended up with my own clothing line. I became preoccupied with imagery—seeing other people dressed up in public and longing to be beautiful one day. I think most little girls play that game, but this was coming from another place.

I would pretend I was extremely "fancy," dressing up and tossing feather boas around my shoulders. I loved gowns and would watch old black-and-white movies, with actresses in stylized clothing and with stylized voices, as a source of inspiration. I loved watching my great-grandmother Reba make clothes on her sewing machine; she was an amazing seamstress, and I could never get over how she could make a piece of material turn into a fashionable suit or dress.

I also relished going to Mama Bird's house in Louisville, my father's hometown, with all its fancy French furniture with curved legs. I imagined myself sitting on it in haute couture. I even loved the over-the-topness of Liberace, thinking he was "beautiful." (On that particular score, my father thought I was crazy. "What the hell is wrong with this child?" he would ask jokingly.)

My mother's mother, Grandmom, would indulge me—with petticoats, with gloves and matching bonnets.

Grandmom indulged me in other ways, too. Whereas my mother wanted me eating vegetables and whole-grain bread, Grandmom fed

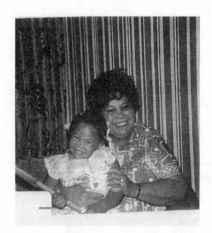

MAMA BIRD (MY FATHER'S MOTHER, ODESSA CLAY) AND LITTLE BIRD (ME).

me the kind of diet that fueled me emotionally, if not so well nutritionally. My grandmother was the first to introduce me to a bowl of Froot Loops, the first to take me to Burger King for cheeseburgers. She used to make me sandwiches with white bread, Miracle Whip, American cheese, and iceberg lettuce.

Food choices were a running battle between my mother and her mother—and a battle inside myself, too, which no doubt added to my difficulties around eating. I knew my mother's food was good for me, but my grandmother's food was too attractive. I had a heightened sensation when I ate it.

No doubt part of that was the love that came with her feeding me. My mother loved me like crazy, of course, and to this day she is my best friend. But she was a young mother and I was her first child, and she thought it was appropriate to take a stern stance. Grandmom, on the other hand, pampered me. She'd let me take long baths in Avon oil, then dry me off and powder me down. Afterward, we'd walk up the street to get a grape soda out of a vending machine, and I'd drink it on her porch while she read me my favorite story—"Cinderella." When she'd take me upstairs for bedtime, she'd offer me water but I'd demand apple juice—and get it. Then she'd

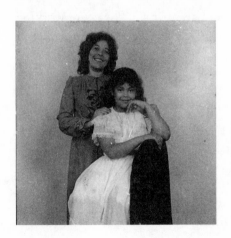

MY MOTHER'S MOTHER, DOROTHY, IS KNOWN AS "THE ROCK" IN OUR FAMILY. SHE BOUGHT ME THAT FLOUNCY DRESS AND INDULGED ME IN OTHER WAYS, TOO.

put on the classical music station. Sometimes we chose jazz, but I generally asked for classical because after having just heard "Cinderella," my imagination would be running wild.

Grandmom had a job as an intake specialist at Berks County Intermediate Unit in Reading, Pennsylvania, which provided various programs and services to area schoolchildren and their parents, and therefore, I, too, wanted to "go to work." I loved putting on her stockings, as she would in the mornings. I would sit there and cross my legs, pretending I was smoking, because she smoked at the time. I actually sneaked to work with her twice, hiding in the back of her car. About ten minutes after she went up to her office, I followed. I loved my grandmom so much, I just had to be near her.

But my mother and I didn't live near my grandmother on a regular basis until we settled on the Main Line when I was four and needed to be in one place so I could attend preschool. Until then, we followed my father around the country, often bouncing between his training camp in Deer Lake, Pennsylvania, another training camp in Miami, and a home he kept in Chicago. And all that bouncing around added up to a pretty chaotic lifestyle, with chaotic eating.

Many kids, by the mid to late 1970s, were not eating in as structured a fashion as their baby-boomer parents had. The era of working moms had taken off in full force, and the ritual of Mom having dinner ready every night promptly at six, with everyone coming to the table, was already falling by the wayside. But eating was more chaotic for me than for most other children.

For instance, at my father's training camp in Pennsylvania, it wasn't my mother who was in charge of the cooking but a woman named Lana Shabazz, who prepared everyone's meals in a communal kitchen, and the trainers and others in my father's entourage would all eat together with us in a communal dining room. So while my mother was trying to keep me on a strict vegan diet, Lana would make steak with mashed potatoes—my favorite. She'd also serve up grits with cheese, and Muslim bean pie, which I loved. I'm not sure exactly what was in it, but it was very sweet, like sweet-potato pie, yet even more delicious.

There was plenty of hotel eating, too. I was in and out of so many hotels and elegantly appointed apartment buildings, in fact, that the first time I walked into my grandmother's front hall, I exclaimed to her, "Grandmom, you have such a little lobby!"

All that feeding by others probably made my mother try to hold the reins on my eating even tighter when she got the chance, and no doubt also contributed to my confusion about what foods were "right," and in what amounts. I was already losing touch with my own internal signals of hunger and satiety because I was busy sam-

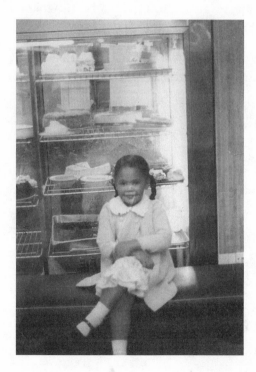

PASTRIES, AND ME SMILING—
NO SURPRISE THERE.

pling so many other people's ideas of what was appropriate foodwise and also always trying to get around my mother's restrictions rather than just eating for eating's sake.

It didn't help that from an early age I never exactly fit in anywhere. I was always straddling two different worlds, never truly belonging to either one. For example, I was raised in a minicommunity of celebrities, but also not. Within my circle was Teddy Jr., of course, as well as Patti LaBelle's son, Zori, and Phillies outfielder Gary Maddox's son, too. But after the age of four or five, I no longer was with my father on a regular basis and, in fact, lived much like other kids in many ways, going to public school some years and so on.

Then, too, I belonged to three different races, which, in a way, plays out as belonging to none. My grandmom and her mom—the one who could sew and whom I also knew well while growing up—are white by all appearances (although there's a bit of Cherokee tucked in), as are my mother's sister and a lot of my cousins. My mother herself is rather unidentifiable racewise; people have asked her if she's everything from South American to Italian to Turkish. And while my father is clearly black and identifies that way, his mother, Mama Bird, had a fair amount of Asian in her; Japanese, specifically.

What it added up to was that people outside my circle generally perceived me as anything but what they were, as "other"—Latino, perhaps, or sometimes even Hawaiian. So I had confusion regarding my racial heritage, which is so central to how people identify themselves in this country. Or, should I say, I had confusion over other people's confusion. I couldn't understand why people were comfortable with the notion of someone having a combined ancestry from different European countries—say, part Irish and part Italian, even if you looked more Italian than Irish—but not a combined ancestry from different continents, in my case, Africa, Europe, and Asia.

In addition, for anyone growing up on Philadelphia's WASPy Main Line, the standard for beauty was fair, with no curves, which I clearly was not going to be.

So I was continuously on the outside looking in, always at a remove from my own circumstances, which creates its own kind of anxiety. And since eating was such a hot-button issue from an early age, food was a natural currency with which I tried to ease the ever-constant dissonance of belonging and not belonging at the same time. I ate to even out my feelings of always being a stranger in my own surroundings.

Making matters more difficult still was other people's reactions to who my father was.

In truth, I didn't start to get a feel for who my father was myself until I was about six. I was browsing through a book we had and turned a page to see a picture of the Beatles lying on the ground in a

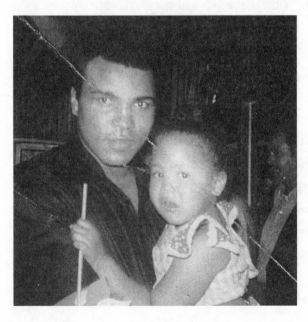

I WAS AROUND
TWO YEARS OLD IN
THIS PICTURE.

boxing ring, with my father standing over them. "Mom," I called out excitedly, "Daddy knows the Beatles!"

"Khaliah," she responded, "they came there to see *him*."

Even then I didn't really get it. All that mattered to me was that my dad had met the Fab Four. (I had the good fortune to meet Ringo a couple of years ago at a fund-raiser. He loved the story.)

Introductions to my father's fame weren't always so benign. When I was in first grade and one of only about two or three kids in the school who were not of strictly European stock, one little girl called out that my father was a draft dodger (it was well known that he was a conscientious objector who refused induction into the army during the Vietnam War) and told me, "Your daddy's nothing but a nigger, anyway." I was also routinely beat up—by boys!—who said I was big and could fight like my father but that they could "take me on." It was a painful way to learn that I was somehow different by virtue of being my father's daughter, particularly because I was a gentle child. I wanted to be seen as feminine, not as a girl who could fight boys.

But it wasn't to be. One day, in fact, about six or seven boys started running at me all at once. They attacked me in the school yard, beating on me and kicking me even after I fell to the ground. "Come on," they kept taunting. "Your dad's Muhammad Ali. You can box. Show us how you can box." My shirt was ripped, and I had a shoe knocked off.

Two teachers finally came over and broke everything up, but one teacher had watched the whole thing with her arms crossed. Clearly, there were adults who were not going to let me feel special. (The next year, and for a few years after that, my parents put me in Friends Select, a private Quaker school in Center City, Philadelphia.)

There were other such instances, too. One day, before I had even started school, I watched Evel Knievel jump the Snake River on television and, deciding that I, too, could accomplish such a feat, rode my bike down thirteen cement steps in front of my grandmother's house. Bloody and bruised, with a broken nose and my forehead swollen over my eyes, I was swept up by my uncle Darren, my mother's brother. As he rushed me off to the emergency room, the lady next door, who had passively watched the whole thing, commented, "That's what the little nigger gets."

Against the backdrop of these difficulties, the drama of my weight continued to play itself out. I would be chosen last for school teams and suffer mortification when it was time to buy gym shorts or other clothes. And I was always dieting or being dieted by my mother one way or another. When I was about eight years old, she sent me to a program near my house called Youth Med. By that point she had made it very clear to me that she felt I was overweight.

Several days each week after school, overweight kids went to get counseling—and to get weighed. I remember feeling very embarrassed, and also terrified at first, not wanting to be there. But after a while, it became a comfort zone. I knew it meant that I was making my mother happy. I could see how dissatisfied she was with me. We would be looking in a catalog and she'd say, "See, you could have a pretty dress like this, or you could have these kinds of clothes, if you looked like that."

Of course, while going to Youth Med was a way of connecting with her, and while she truly meant her words to be encouraging, the whole setup added to my negative feelings about myself. I remember thinking, "Well, I must not be pretty. Something's wrong with me." I felt really ugly.

Other adults in my circle could see the dynamic, and tried in their own way to help. One was Teddy's mother. She never tried to get between my mother and me regarding eating, but as a large woman herself, she simply embraced me as I was without ever intimating that I needed to be "made over." Her warmth was a great comfort to me.

I also remember another large woman, a neighbor of my grandmother's named Mina Williford, who went so far as to try to take an active role. She told me, "You're a big girl. You're always going to be fat. Give it up." She fed me dishes like fried bananas, and while I loved her acceptance of my size, her complacency about my weight only made me more resistant to the idea that it would forever be a part of who I was. I said to myself, even at age eight, "Someday, this is not going to be."

So I worked really hard at Youth Med, losing eight, maybe even ten, pounds, regularly eating my fruits and vegetables and all that.

Youth Med saw an opportunity in me, and with my mother's permission promoted itself on local television with the news that Muhammad Ali's daughter was slimming down on its program. There I was doing sit-ups with a cameraman two feet away from me, breathing too heavily, my face contorted.

I also appeared on *People Are Talking* with Tom Bergeron. James Coco and I were the "fat" guests, talking about our eating problems.

Then came a call from the *Today* show. On one hand, the idea of going on national television, live, was horrifying—more pressure than I thought I could bear. Also, I was absolutely overwhelmed by the idea of being interviewed by Jane Pauley. She seemed so wonderful and perfect; I thought she was the most beautiful thing ever, and I wanted nothing more than to be like her. I used to wake up in the morning as a small child and watch the *Today* show just to see her. *That* was my Sesame Street.

On the other hand, I was mature and articulate, for a kid, and relished the chance to meet her.

I remember how scared I was the morning of the show. I so didn't want to disappoint her. But she was amazing—gentle and very sweet. And she was so genuinely caring. I was terribly nervous, but she made me feel very much at ease. I had an extremely warm feeling from her.

She was pregnant at the time, which only heightened the glow she radiated.

The interview with Jane Pauley actually strengthened my resolve. I remember thinking, if I somehow manage to keep dieting, this could be my reality—to be beautiful and powerful, to be able to help others. This is why you have to stick to your diet, I reasoned hard with myself. This is what you could be like someday.

But a nine-year-old's determination is no match for her circumstances. I gained back the weight I had lost. I remember feeling that dieting was a losing battle. I would think, okay, this low-calorie food is fine for today, but what about tomorrow? Tomorrow, there's going to be braised beef and rice for lunch at school, and I'm going to want that. It was like an alcoholic not wanting to fall off the wagon but preparing to, anyway. I would actually pray to God to help me slim down.

After I gained back the weight, I joined Weight Watchers. This was on my own. My mother didn't discourage me, but she didn't push it. Once a week, I'd take a long walk alone to a dingy church basement with those collapsible metal chairs. It was summer, and it was hot, and even though by this time I was already an experienced dieter and knew the drill, while I was going through the paces I felt I couldn't handle it. I was the only kid there, and I was miserable. I remember coming home from one meeting and putting some tuna fish on a small piece of bread. I sat down and bit into it and thought, okay, I can do this. But then time passed and I was eating again. The food just didn't hold me. So I'd make these awful sandwiches with white bread, bologna, mayonnaise, and cheese, and a tall glass of orange juice. Or I'd heat up a package of ramen noodles. I'd wonder, how am I ever going to get on top of this? I was hungry, and I literally recall thinking to myself that my life was going to be hell.

I ended up losing only a pound or two. It was just too much responsibility for a grade-schooler. On top of that, I was probably reacting on some level to my mother's obsession with not being overweight precisely by overeating. It was as if they were two directly opposing forces.

For all that, I kept trying, but the effort was scattered and haphazard. For instance, when the ice-cream truck came, I knew to get a Fudgsicle or a Creamsicle instead of ice cream because my mother told me they had fewer calories. But what's that in the face of unstructured eating—and lots of it—at other times?

Although not conscious of my motive at the time, I tried to compensate for my failure at dieting, at looking pretty, by being really good—courteous as well as nurturing. If a kid was crying in the playground, I was the one to comfort her. I remember one little girl with Down's syndrome playing in a park near my grandmother's house. She fell down and was bleeding, and no one would touch her, as if she had germs. I ran over to help her.

I was always trying to please adults, too, seeking their approval through deeds if not through looks. I had a terrible fear of displeasing people (which is still an issue with me today), so I tried always to be very well behaved and respectful to my elders. If I spent the night at a friend's house, I would make her bed as well as my own. If there was a piece of trash in the street, I would pick it up.

I also felt, on a conscious level, that by leaving adults delighted with my manners, I was making my father's light look even brighter. I saw myself in a way as his ambassador, and that, in turn, made me feel closer to him.

The irony of it was that my father's acceptance of my appearance was unconditional. He was definitely one of those daddies who always made his little girl feel beautiful. He never once made me conscious of my weight, instead making a point of telling me how good-looking I was, how pretty I was. He is probably one of the very few people in my life who told me that in a way that I believed it.

But his influence on my daily life was sparse. While I was with him frequently before I started school, once my mother and I set up house near Philadelphia, I saw him only a few times a year, in part because we were far away from each other but also because my parents' relationship gradually dissolved. On one level it was not different from what other children go through when their parents drift apart and one of them lives somewhere else. But because of who my father was, he always had so many people competing for his attention that it was harder for me to ever have him to myself. His life, even more than that of many other celebrities, was not his own. Even the day I was born, he was giving a press conference about the upcoming "Rumble in the Jungle" fight with George Foreman, in which he regained his heavyweight title, and missed the actual birth.

Those times when he was able to be with me, it wasn't the way other children could be with their fathers. I remember one incident in

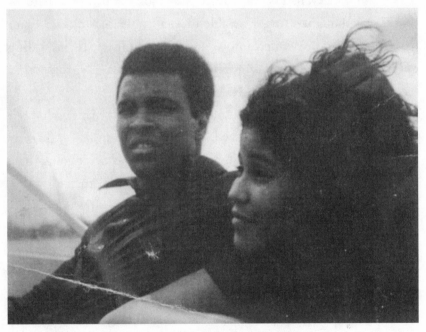

A RARE PHOTO OF MY PARENTS TOGETHER.

which my father came to see me play the cello in my school orchestra. I had gotten quite good, to the point that I dreamed about becoming a classical music conductor, although admittedly, that, too, was about wanting to look good. To me, to be a conductor was to be beautiful, and when I played music, in my head I was thin and willowy.

But as excited as I was that my father came to see me, his presence created such a stir that it sort of took over the concert, and by the time it came to my solo, I was so flummoxed that I had forgotten all my music and had to make something up as the orchestra leader turned directly toward me. It was a blur of trying so hard to impress my father, to look good to him, yet with the background "noise" of his celebrity confounding me so that I couldn't perform at my best.

Unfortunately, my father rarely, if ever, got to see me perform at other times, and not just musically. I also worked to excel at riding horses and, in fact, had become such a good jumper by my early teens that it was thought I might be able to qualify for the Junior Olympics. Riding, too, was tied into a notion of thinness. In my riding outfits—jodhpurs, boots, and hat—I was someone else, someone I felt very good about.

But my father's absence ate at me, and to cope I ate my way through not seeing him regularly. I realized, too, after a certain point, that my parents weren't ever going to be together, that he was never going to be in my life in an everyday way, which only added to my frustration that things with me were not the way I wanted them to be. It was a kind of anger and despair that, looking back, I suppose I tried to quell with food.

It was making my mother more and more anxious, to the point that she set up an appointment with my pediatrician specifically to talk about my weight. What he said on that visit was shocking—to both of us.

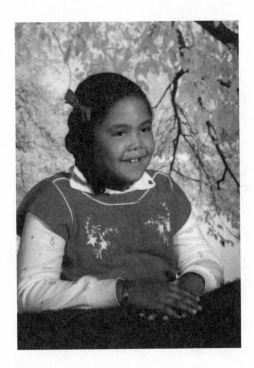

FOURTH GRADE, AROUND THE TIME
I WENT ON THE *TODAY* SHOW WHILE
DIETING ON YOUTH MED.

"Leave her alone. She's fine." His theory was that if you put children on diets, you start a lifetime of emotional problems, of complications. Besides, he said, although I was chubby, I was also big-boned and appropriately pudging up in that prepubescent way a lot of kids do before their final growth spurt in adolescence. Leave my eating to its own devices, he felt, and I'd end up at a weight that would be healthy for me.

To this day a part of me believes that if my mother had listened to my doctor's advice, I would have slimmed down on my own. Perhaps I wouldn't have turned out trim, but I would have ended up a very respectable size twelve. I don't think my weight would have followed me so tenaciously.

But my mother's reaction was, "Absolutely not. Look at her." And so the cycle continued, with me feeling something was wrong with me for not being able to control my eating and my mother trying her best to control my eating by herself. "Are you really going to have that?" she would ask. "That's not good for you. That's not going to help you."

One time, maybe it was the year before I turned ten, I came downstairs one Christmas morning to find a teen dieting book under the tree. I wasn't insulted. I was excited, although the gift also gave me knots in my stomach because of that overwhelming sense that I couldn't do this. The feeling was heightened by a picture of a girl on the cover who had really skinny legs. It created that same kind of anticipation and anxiety I would get every time I started a diet.

The weight chart in the book said I should weigh 88 pounds. At the time, I weighed 114. But there was a prescribed eating and exercise plan and I felt, as I had already felt many times before, that if I could just call up the willpower to follow it, I'd reach my goal.

I went to bed happy that night. It was as if just by reading the book I was already making myself thinner.

Then Christmas vacation gave way to New Year's, school soon started again, and not long after I was up to 120.

2

BAD TO WORSE

ometime between the fourth and fifth grade I was officially diagnosed with dyslexia. I had always known something was wrong, or different, and so did my teachers. I was one of those kids whose mothers are told as early as their child is in first grade, "She's very bright. She's just not applying herself."

I probably don't just have dyslexia. There's a strong chance that I also have attention deficit disorder, or at least some attributes of ADD, even if I don't meet the clinical definition. But at the time I was put through that whole battery of tests kids go through to figure out what's wrong, ADD wasn't being explored as consistently as it is today. Girls, in particular, were thought not to have it, since at that point it was pretty much always paired with hyperactivity, which is more of a boy thing than a girl thing. It wasn't as well established that you could have ADD without the hyper component.

Being labeled with a learning disability did not feel good. It seemed like I was embarking on yet another endless struggle to add to the struggle of my weight.

On another level, however, the diagnosis was a relief. From a very young age I had difficulty concentrating while reading, and writing did not come easily to me, and this explained why. At the same time, I was well-spoken, and the diagnosis helped me realize that I had been relying on the spoken word to make up for my trouble communicating—and being communicated with—on paper. In short, I had cultivated an articulateness beyond my years and was playing to my strength. I think that's why people like Jane Pauley so impressed me. She was a great speaker, and even by the time I met her, I had intuited that speaking was something I was going to need to be good at.

Once the diagnosis was confirmed, my parents transferred me to a school for children with learning disabilities called the Woodren School. This was now my third elementary school. To complicate matters still more, out of a small class of about half a dozen kids, I was one of only two girls, the other of whom was as tall as I was chubby, even though it was I who was usually the tallest girl in class.

Despite the difficulties, I had wonderful relationships with my teachers at Woodren. I got along well with my classmates, too. Some were just plain nice, and others thought it was cool that my father was who he was. By that time I thought it was pretty cool, too, although that kind of status is a double-edged sword. It gets you "in," but it often leaves you not knowing whether you really belong.

For instance, while some classmates and their parents just treated me like a person, other families would invite me to dinner, and then their neighbors would happen to breeze through for no particular reason and say hi. As the only child of color in the school, I wondered whether my popularity in those cases was the result of being "the right kind of black" because of my father's celebrity, the way the bigoted pizza parlor owner's son in *Do the Right Thing* says someone like Magic Johnson, Eddie Murphy, or Prince is "no nigger" because of his vaunted status.

I didn't have much time to focus on that in a conscious way, though, as there was an even bigger shift in my life at that time than the shift in schools. My mother and I had moved in with a new man in her life—Kenny Gamble, of Gamble and Huff music. Kenny and his partner, Leon Huff, wrote and/or produced so many hits, including "If You Don't Know Me By Now," "Me and Mrs. Jones," "I'm Gonna Make You Love Me," and "Back Stabbers," and Kenny lived a lifestyle that reflected his success. Our own house, while in a perfectly pleasant, even upper-class, suburb, was modest. Kenny's was a twenty-nine-room mansion, a huge brick affair set well back from the road behind a wrought-iron gate. He had a housekeeper, fresh flowers at all times, a thirty-foot dining room, and all the other accoutrements of wealth.

But that wasn't what made living with Kenny Gamble—"Luqman" to everyone who knows him—so wonderful. It was that we were family, and he was truly a day-to-day father to me. Just as important, my mother's love for him was strong and passionate, and he made her feel very secure. I had never seen her so happily in love before because my parents' relationship was over before I would have been old enough for such feelings to register.

My mother had actually first met Luqman (LUKE-mahn) when she was a girl of nine or ten. Her godmother had a club in south Jersey called the High Hat, where she cooked great food and new talent would come to showcase their music. Kenny Gamble would come there to sing with his group, the Romeos.

Then, as a young adult, my mother met him again. Living near

Philly and knowing Teddy Pendergrass, who was one of the people in Luqman's musical circle, it was bound to happen.

For years the two were just good friends, talking for hours and hours, really communicating. But over time the warmth of their friendship turned into a very serious relationship. My mother's time with my father had been serious, too, but she was so young when they were together. This was the first relationship in which she really felt like a woman. And they truly lived as a couple under one roof. Luqman wasn't traveling all the time, like my father was.

For me, living with Uncle Luqman was pure heaven. Every day at his house was the best day of my life. We'd all have dinner together every night. We'd take walks after we ate. He'd take me for long car rides—we'd eat turkey sandwiches on rye—and we'd talk politics, we'd talk God. It was so wonderful I wasn't even hungry for the food I was eating. I even slimmed down some.

Life at Luqman's house could get very exciting, in wonderful ways. Big musical talent, or at least up-and-coming talent, would always be passing through—Whitney Houston, the O'Jays, Stephanie Mills, and most important of all to me, Dionne Warwick, whose music, even when I was a child, always brought me to tears and goose bumps. When I hear her rendition of "Alfie" or "Moments Aren't Moments," I am transported—there's no other way to put it.

I had actually met Dionne Warwick as a little girl, when my mother and I stayed at Teddy Pendergrass's house for a while. She used to come over and play pool. But neither there nor at Uncle Luqman's could I bring myself to try to have a conversation with her, as talkative as I was. I was so in awe of her that I couldn't bear it, and also didn't want to crowd her space. My respect kept me from risking making a pest of myself.

But soon my awkwardness around her would be the least of my concerns. About two years into our stay at Luqman's, another woman came into his life, and my mother wasn't willing to share. She had, quite frankly, been down that road with my father, and older now with some life experience under her belt and a stronger sense of self, she left, and we returned to our house on the Main Line. In Mia Farrow fashion, my mother took a goldfish from Luqman's house and nothing else, although he offered to give her a car and do whatever else he could to make the transition easier materially.

Uncle Luqman continued to be a father figure to me, even though we no longer lived together as a family. These days, we don't talk often, but he was there for the birth of my son, and he is there for me if I ever need him. Further to his credit, he was always concerned about my weight, not in a shallow way but because he was afraid about how it might affect my health. "You're a beautiful girl," he used to tell me when I eventually grew to my largest. "You're beautiful either way, but this isn't good for you."

Still, despite the warm feelings even to this day, when my mother and I moved out of Luqman's house, life as we had come to know and appreciate it soon came crashing down around us. One of the many casualties of that crash was my eating habits. I was now back to overeating at meals, overeating between meals, eating haphazardly instead of sitting down to meals, and so on. The depressing feeling of that wonderful period of my life coming to an abrupt end was ever present, and I was trying to fill the void with food.

An aspect of the situation that only added to making healthful living too hard to accomplish was that my mother soon met someone else, someone I felt didn't treat her well enough. Along with him, younger siblings were now in the picture—my brother, Jared, and my sister, Jenna.

They are both blessings to me, and the three of us are all very close, but soon after Jenna was born, the situation became truly desperate in that my mother began to suffer flare-ups of lupus that really got the better of her. It was suspected that she had lupus even while she was a teenager, and she was officially diagnosed with the disease in 1978, when I was four years old, but it had remained under wraps for the better part of ten years. (I suspect part of the reason she had gone through such a strict vegan phase, besides trying to keep down her weight, was to attempt to get a handle on her illness by eating as much as possible with her health in mind.)

What the severe lupus flare-ups meant in practical terms was that by the age of thirteen, I was doing a lot of parenting. (My siblings' father was not what you would call reliable.) My mother was sometimes so sick that she couldn't get out of bed, which left me to get myself ready for school and tend to my siblings as best as possible before I left for the day, dressing them, telling them stories, and feeding them breakfast.

I felt, in a way, parentless—and scared. Here my mother was with a debilitating disease, and it wasn't too long before that my father had been officially diagnosed with Parkinson's. I had always bought into the resilient, boundless energy that was around him, but at the same time, I was aware for years that there were neurological problems. Now there was no denying it, and it was both parents whose lives were in the balance with serious health concerns. Making it even more complicated and confusing was that by this time I was fully aware of who my father was, so that he loomed large not just for me but in general, yet he wasn't there, at least not on any consistent basis. It's extremely disquieting to know you have a parent who is ever present yet, for all practical purposes, absent.

That realization, in the midst of tough circumstances, made me eat even more. It was a typical pattern of overweight people: I'd go to school not hungry because I'd eaten so much the night before (it's not like there was a family dinnertime; eating went on all evening), then I'd be ravenous by lunch and unable to control my portions, starting the whole overeating cycle again.

There were other stresses contributing to my low state, too. One was that I had a couple of my own life-threatening bouts with illness. When I was twelve or thirteen, my mother sent me to a horseback riding camp. At the end of the season, a camp counselor assigned me to clean out a pregnant horse's stall, and the horse kicked and bit me. Soon after, I started to have pains in my neck. I couldn't bear light in my eyes. A spinal tap confirmed that I had encephalitis—a serious illness in which the lining of the brain becomes inflamed—and I was in the hospital for weeks. (I came out of the hospital thirteen pounds thinner than when I went in. As sick as I had been, I was thrilled about that.)

Sometime after, perhaps because my immune system had not fully come back yet, I came down with viral meningitis and was bedridden for close to two months. I didn't just miss a lot of school but was out of commission all ways round. I then developed mononucleosis, which put me behind that much further.

On top of all the illnesses—mine, my mother's, and my father's—around the time I reached adolescence, my mother took my father to court for child support. Like many couples with children who split up, mine had issues over money. The sad truth is that we were strapped financially. It might seem hard to fathom, given who my father is, but by that time he had had other women and other children and, like so many dads who aren't on the scene, competing attentions that caused his prioritizing to be arranged in a different way from what might have been expected.

Part and parcel of that is that people like my father have handlers and others to manage their money. That is, celebrities are in certain ways often removed from the details of their finances, so although they are technically in charge, it can be harder for them to stay on top of whether their money is being channeled in exactly the ways they might think appropriate if left to make such decisions by themselves.

The court battle dragged on for years, and carrying around the tension of the lawsuit, I ate my way through it. I continued to eat my way through the other stresses as well, and by that time, so did my mother and my brother, who was old enough by then to have out-of-control food habits. We had become a fat family. Food was our refuge, as well as our entertainment. As in so many other American households, every eating occasion was a minivacation from stress, an opportunity to defuse tension, to cope. And the eating was chaotic, not family centered.

It's not that my mother never made an effort for us to all sit down together to a meal. Sometimes she'd try very hard. But with her own illness and her own tension taking its toll, more often than not each of us would eat whatever we found in the house when we felt like eating. My mother's own weight ballooned not just because of that but also because of the increasing steroid dosages she was forced to take to quell the lupus. Her eating truly was no longer her own.

Ironically, through this entire period I did have normal teenager moments. I would still manage to spend time on the phone, like teens do, obsessing with my friends over the things that newly adolescent girls obsess over. I didn't go to the mall with them, or to parties or dances, but I at least kept myself on the periphery of a social loop. I even helped with the construction of a Habitat for Humanity house as part of a school project and thought about becoming a candy striper. My grandmother had by this point started doing some part-time work as a home health aide to earn a little extra money on the side, and I felt that by becoming a candy striper, I would be following in her footsteps. But I was too young, and really couldn't have carved out the time to indulge myself in that kind of volunteer work, anyway.

I managed to "volunteer" in another way, however, by taking on a guidance-counselor-like role with my classmates. I was the one everyone else came to with their problems. I liked it. It allowed me to be with people my own age, yet kept the focus off me and my own troubles. As teenagers, my classmates were only too glad to have someone who would listen to their concerns, not thinking about the fact that as the fat girl, I wasn't experiencing firsthand the very things on which they would seek my advice—dating, clothes, and all that. Or maybe they *were* conscious of the fact that I was somewhat "outside," which made them more comfortable to share secrets with me that they would have been embarrassed to share with people who had higher status in our social circle.

Either way, being part of a crowd, even in that tenuous fashion, was a kind of adrenaline for me. It kept me feeling on top of things, like I had a handle on things—except eating. Nothing stopped me from eating, although not for lack of trying. I'd lose ten pounds, then gain twenty; lose twenty, then gain forty. Cabbage diet, raw food diet, more Weight Watchers, plain old starvation—I yo-yoed through all of them, up and down, up and down, with the spikes of the "ups" always outdoing the "downs." (I hated the mean girls, the ones you find in every single middle school across America, yet envied their bodies and the way the boys tripped over themselves trying to get their attention.)

Losing weight under my circumstances would have been hard no matter what, but I think part of my difficulty was that while I was always there to lend an ear to others, I had no one to talk to myself. My father was unreachable, and I didn't want to upset my mother. So I stuffed my feelings through stuffing food; I was shoving them all deep in—internalizing, as therapists say, rather than getting any of it off my chest and away from me.

I was exhausted, too. In addition to going to school and helping to take care of my brother and sister, by the time I was thirteen, I was working. It was easy to get jobs because my height and my build belied my age; I could pass for fifteen, and simply used a different last name to avoid any suspicion.

I started out babysitting, but over time I would take on sort of a nanny role—cleaning and getting dinner ready for a family before the parents arrived home from work. I was constantly falling asleep on my feet—pitching in at home, going to school, and then going to a job before getting back to the house. I'd also have to tend to chores like raking leaves in the fall and shoveling snow in the winter. When a household doesn't have a man, or a man you can count on, no one's going to do those things if you don't. In a bad snowstorm, my mother would put on her boots and start shoveling the driveway, and when she got tired it was my turn. It was that simple.

The thing is, when you have so many responsibilities that you're constantly overhwhelmingly tired, you eat in an effort to rouse yourself out of your stupor, to try to dispel the tedium of going through the motions while your body sags from fatigue. I'd feed my siblings, then sit there and finish up their plates after they left the table.

There were times I would cry myself to sleep. But at the same time, I was determined—determined not to depend on my father's money, determined to be independent rather than vulnerable to having the rug pulled out from under me.

So, along with my babysitting jobs, I also had a lucrative (for a child) jewelry business as well as a perfume business. I made earrings at a local crafts store—long, dangly, earthy-looking earrings with cobalt and red beads—and sold them at Teddy's mother's shop. She owned a hairdressing salon at which she had a clientele that consisted of lawyers, judges, even local entertainment figures like ballet dancers, and she let me display them there. I also sold perfumes at Teddy's mother's shop by buying empty bottles in bulk, then mixing natural oils with other scents.

Just about all of the money I earned I gave directly to my mother, which was okay with me. While I was determined not to have to depend on anyone, I was more and more depressed—and ever fatter—

and less and less interested in the usual adolescent preoccupation of buying clothes and makeup. Normally, when you're a teenager, even a fat one, you entertain notions of unfolding into a glorious creature who sparkles, who turns heads when she enters a room; you know you're not a finished product. But by that point I was so tired and so beaten that I often *felt* finished. It was hard to imagine myself in a better future.

It showed. I kept wearing the same drab-colored tentlike outfits to cover me, which only made me look heavier. My grandmother would always be saying, "Where do we find husky clothes for Lilah?" (an endearing pet name she had for me), but hearing the words *husky* or *big girl*, I would just want to crawl into a hole and die. The last thing that made me want to do was shop—or leave a store with a shopping bag that said 16-PLUS.

One time, however, my grandmother took matters into her own hands. She drove over from Reading and just totally cleaned me up—took me to the hairdresser's (they made my hair cascade in

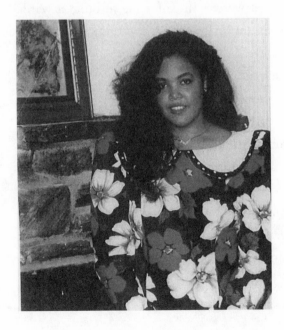

READY FOR MY FIRST, AND ONLY, SCHOOL DANCE AT AGE SIXTEEN. I WAS EXTREMELY UNCOMFORTABLE ABOUT GOING.

beautiful curls) and bought me a whole new outfit. It was camel-colored stirrup pants with a matching V-neck, cable-knit sweater that buttoned. Underneath, I wore a coral-colored blouse. I was thrilled. Not only had someone taken the time to make me look prettier, but also, the sweater covered my thighs and behind in just the right way, minimizing all the widest points. I knew very clearly with that outfit that fashion could change the way a woman felt about herself, that it could make her happy, and I tucked that away for use later on when consulting on the designs for my own line of clothes.

At the time, however, in the there and then, what counted was that when I went into school dressed like that, the popular group called me over. "Khaliah, come sit with us. Be with us." That made me feel great. But by the same token, it also poured gasoline into the fire of my discontent with myself. It made me feel all the more that I was never going to be able to get on top of my weight, that I was holding on to something slippery and would fall.

Besides, what was I going to do, wear the same outfit to school every day? The resources just weren't there for me to build a wardrobe, and even if they were, my shame about my body would have kept me from filling my closet.

In the midst of my despair, I was given the good fortune to be tapped as a cohost of a show on Black Entertainment Television called *Teen Summit*. My mother, through her connections in the entertainment world, led me to the people who helped me secure the spot. It was one of those shows during which young adolescents talk about issues of the day.

I wasn't very good at it. While I was thrilled for the opportunity, I wasn't ready for it, especially with all that was going on in my life. And I was always very uncomfortable and self-conscious about the way I looked, which got in the way of my being a warm host who could help guests feel at ease and bring out the best in themselves.

But I *was* entrepreneurial, if not happy with my body, and the experience gave me an idea.

I picked up the phone and called NBC, ABC, and CBS in Los Angeles, said whose daughter I was, and managed to get appointments with executives at NBC and CBS. I had never tried using my father's name to open doors before, so I was extremely nervous. But arriving in California after five days on a Trailways bus, I mustered the courage to tell them I thought the time was ripe for a national show with human-interest topics, like Oprah's, but with teens as the focus. I wanted not only to cover various issues but have the show be a resource, too, empower teens with information on where they could go to get tested for HIV, for instance, where they could go if they became pregnant.

They listened respectfully and treated me well, telling me that they liked me and felt I was compelling. But they said, in no uncertain terms, that they weren't convinced teens would watch a talk show, so there'd be no guarantee of an audience and therefore advertisers would be hesitant to come on board. It was a hard lesson. My father's name could *open* doors, but not ensure that I'd get to walk through them.

A year and a half later, Rikki Lake was hosting a show much like the one I had proposed. By then, of course, I had long since returned east, to my life of school and work and taking care of my family. I had also essentially reached my adult height and was now pushing two hundred pounds.

3

THE CINDERELLA
YEARS

MUHAMMAD ALI'S DAUGHTER, KHALIAH,
FLOATS INTO THE AMERICAN SPORTCASTERS
AWARD DINNER ON THE ARM OF HER FATHER.

can't find the clipping, but the quote in a New York newspaper
went something like that.

It was my Cinderella moment. After years of not quite estrange-
ment but a relationship that had been very much strained, I was now
sixteen and old enough to make my own plans to see my father, at least
sometimes. The event he took me to was a gala affair studded with a
veritable Who's Who of sports and media figures mixed with financial
moguls.

I rode the train up from Philadelphia to New York in a budget-
blowing outfit I had bought for the occasion—a tunic-length jacket

heavily embroidered with gold, a black skirt with three rhinestone buttons, and high heels. The jacket covered all the things I didn't want people to see and also had a princess seam, which meant it came from under the breast down to the waist, making it seem fitted, not boxy. The skirt was A-line. My aim with those cuts was to hide my heft a little, give myself a more flattering silhouette.

But as uncomfortable as I was about the state of my body, and as nervous as I was about being introduced to such a rarefied circle of people that evening, I relished every moment of my first exposure to such a large and glamorous sphere of notables. And I loved, absolutely loved, being brought out that way as my father's daughter.

Then the clock, so to speak, struck twelve. Some of my father's handlers said there was no room for me at his hotel, I was left on my own, and I walked in my heels to New York's Penn Station to catch the 1:32 A.M. train back to Philly. I had just enough money, down to the penny, for my ticket.

As deflating as that was, however, something changed that night. There was more out there, and now I had gotten a taste of it.

Thus began what I call my Cinderella years, the years of getting to dress up once in a while and go to the "ball," but mostly existing hemmed in by the all-too-real circumstances of my own life—a shortage of money, a sick mother, two younger siblings, and then a third, Lydia. It was all inextricably wrapped together with my weight and my inability to find the emotional or physical energy to do much about it.

While I worked at helping my mother make ends meet and take care of the younger children, I never looked at the intermittent invitations to attend functions in New York merely as fairy tale fluff, as fleeting reprieves from my situation. I used each new exposure to those among the country's top power brokers as an opportunity for an amazing education.

For instance, through the president of the American Sportcasters Association, Lou Schwartz, I was made a spokesperson for the "Say No to Drugs, Yes to Education" campaign, and being in that position helped lead to black-tie dinners during which I'd watch some of the hugest people in the world—Ted Turner, Oliver Stone, Arthur Ashe—talk to audiences on subjects they felt passionate about. In listening, I was learning about speech making, about rallying people around a cause or an idea. I didn't know how I'd use my newfound knowledge, but I had a clear sense that what I was learning and the contacts I was making would bear fruit later.

At times I even had the opportunity to enter into one-on-one conversations with people in positions of political as well as financial power, including former New York City mayor David Dinkins and then-mayor Rudy Giuliani.

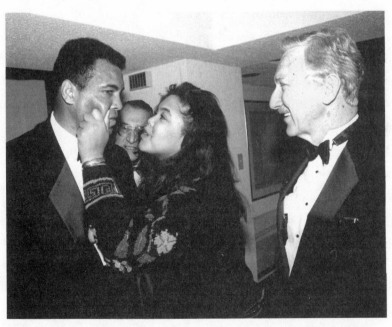

MY FATHER AND I JUST BEFORE A BLACK TIE EVENT FOR THE AMERICAN SPORTSCASTERS ASSOCIATION. LOU SCHWARTZ IS ON THE RIGHT. Courtesy American Sportscasters Association.

At the end of a formal-attire evening or other mixing with influential figures, the other half of my dual life would kick in. True to coach-into-pumpkin form, I would leave the party earlier than the other guests and take the cheapest transportation back to Philly, either a train or bus, and work an 11 P.M. to 7 A.M. shift as, say, a nursing home attendee or home health aide. As much as my schoolwork (and school attendance) suffered, it was a logical choice for someone with a family in financial need, as my grandmother had been doing that kind of moonlighting, and my mother had begun the same kind of work, too.

But also, I thought night work would be a great dieting opportunity because it left me too tired to eat during the day and too busy, I reasoned, to eat during the graveyard shift. I was wrong. A fat person can always manage to carve out time to eat—too much. The hunger doesn't rest.

I also worked evenings for telemarketing firms and catalog companies, but both types of work proved dyslexic nightmares. I'd send out the wrong orders, lose my job, and move on to another company. It finally caught up with me. A supervisor at one place would speak to his or her counterpart at another in deciding whether to take me on and be told, "Yup, I remember her. I fired her."

Another type of work I did to help pay bills was nannying. For one particular family, I nannied one summer from 8 A.M. to 6 P.M., five days a week. They had a little baby I tended to all day—and I ate and ate while caring for her. I even started bringing food to the house. By the time I quit, I was up to 270 pounds.

I had tried to counter my eating by taking long hot walks with the baby in the stroller. And at first I'd be mildly successful in my attempts, losing up to 10 or even 15 pounds at a time. But then I'd put it all back on again. It was a pattern that would repeat itself often. I ranged from the mid 200s to about 270 for years.

Weight aside, I could bear the seemingly endless days and nights of drudgery and exhaustion because I knew something exciting was bound to be around the corner. The fairy godmother of fate would come, and I'd get invited to an event. And that, in turn, would give me an opportunity to network so that I could work at turning fate into activities of my own making.

I was, in other words, laying the groundwork to build a professional life. Sometimes I'd even get a paid spokesperson gig, which would help tide us over a little more comfortably for a few weeks. At one point I was given the opportunity to host a television show much like the one I had pitched out in L.A. An education vehicle for UPN-Viacom, it was called *Rappin'* and aired regionally in the Philadelphia area, D.C., Delaware, and parts of New Jersey.

The format of the show was for me to introduce about a dozen teenagers sitting around on blocks to both entertainers and other guests who could speak with them about serious subjects affecting their lives. For example, we had the mayor of Cherry Hill, New Jersey, come once to talk about education issues. My role was to help the teens and the guests connect a little more informally than they might have been able to in a different venue.

I was never sure whether I was any good at it. But the show won the Pennsylvania Broadcasters Award, and I was nominated for a regional Emmy, so I have to assume that I did okay.

A couple of other validating experiences also occurred during my later teen years, experiences that touched me more deeply than any award could have. They involved my father.

One time the two of us were walking down a hallway together. He was carrying his championship belt from one of his fights with Joe Frazier. It was a wide green leather piece with a huge gold medallion in the center that had the initials WBC (World Boxing Championship), the kind of thing you keep with your trophies and other awards. He had it with him for a photo shoot or something, and I asked if I could hold it. He immediately handed it to me and said, "You keep it. You're going to carry my name on, you're going to do the right thing. It's yours." I was so choked up I could hardly breathe.

Another time, he and I were sitting around a table with lawyers and handlers talking about the possibility of my being able to dip into some kind of trust fund. The meeting wasn't going well—the object of some of his financial advisers seemed to be to give me as little as possible and make it as difficult as possible for me to have access to it. Finally, after hours of back-and-forth, during which my father remained largely quiet, he took my hand under the table and slipped a ring on my finger.

I immediately went to take it off. My father's motion was so abrupt in the midst of all the belabored proceedings that he actually startled me, and my automatic gesture was to try to "undo" the bit of flurry. But he grabbed my arm firmly and stuck the ring back on. "Fuck 'em," he said. "Sell it or keep it. Do what you have to do. Take this ring and go. It's yours."

It was a flawless ruby, between five and six carats. Whether he had been planning on giving it to me when the meeting was all over, or whether he had even originally planned for me to have it at all, I'll never know. I just know I would never sell it.

The ring incident happened not long after the protracted suit between my parents came to an end. I think, in part, it might have been my father's way of saying that while he and my mother had split up, a father and daughter never could. But ironically, only a year or so ago, when I was already into my thirties, my mother told me that even at the height of the case, which at times had become very contentious, she and my father would talk, and that at one point, he actually asked her to marry him.

"Mom," I questioned. "How could he ask you to marry him after all that had gone on?"

"Love is like water, Khaliah," she answered. "It seeps through everything. You can't stop it. Even the Bible says so."

Close to the time my father gave me the ring, I enrolled in Rosemont College, a small Catholic girls' school about ten miles outside of Philadelphia. I had to talk the director of admissions into letting me in, as my grades had never been very good.

I decided to major in political science, but my very first poly-sci professor in freshman year told me, "You're not going to last here. You will never graduate from this or any other college. As long as you're here, you're welcome. But for what you're going to accomplish in life, college is not a relevant path."

I was boiling. True, my high school grades were far from promising, but I so wanted an education. How could he speak to me like that?

He was right, though. It was only a couple of years later that I was helping to run a campaign to elect to Congress a man named Joe Hoeffel, a Pennsylvania Democrat. He appointed me director of minority and student affairs. I was also picked by Pennsylvania's Montgomery County Democratic Party chair Marcel Groen for consulting work. These politicians didn't come to me. I went to the Democratic Party to offer my services. By then I had been to enough black-tie events and had met enough movers and shakers to hold my own among successful people, and I wanted to put to work the things I felt I had learned—facilitating, convincing, bringing people together.

In my freshman year itself, my confidence was bolstered by the fact that while I was living at the dorm, I lost thirty pounds—without even expending too much effort.

I wasn't that far from home, never that far from the difficulties my mother was going through, and always there to pitch in if things became too difficult for her to handle by herself. But I think that being away from my house, creating my own life apart from my family, must have loosened the hold on my hunger, on my need to "stuff" all the time.

My mother thought I looked so good she said I could be a plus-size model, and wanted to send some pictures to modeling agencies. I thought she was crazy but let her take a bunch of black-and-white photos of me with an Instamatic camera. (She thought black-and-white was artier.) Her plan was to get copies to Ford, Wilhelmina, and one or two other top modeling agencies. But when I saw the photos, I was horrified. I wouldn't dare let her send them in. All I could think about was how fat I looked—not simply "big" yet still taut, the way plus-size models tended to look at the time, but fat.

I was all the more keenly aware of how I looked to the outside world because traveling up to New York for events, I was often surrounded by ultrathin, ultrafashionable beautiful people who set the bar for magazine-level beauty. The Philly suburbs were only a hundred miles away, but they were a whole different world, and they had a whole different standard for looking good. At home I may have been perceived as a sweet large girl in a black top and gray skirt. In New York, my looks wouldn't have even registered.

Soon none of that would matter, though. Life got in the way again—seriously. My mother's lupus once more took over her body, and I had to quit college and move back home to help keep things together.

Along with doing work for home-health-aide agencies, I contracted privately with some families, which led to experiences that were particularly degrading. One family would talk within earshot about how I was going to steal things from their house and also called me their "hula girl." (At that point I had long, thick, somewhat wavy hair to my waist—the higher my weight went, the more I would try to hide myself behind my hair.) Another family told me not to eat off their dishes. To cope, I focused on the money I needed to make, even working through Christmas one or two years because working holidays meant being paid overtime.

For all that, however, I suffered an even worse indignity at home. My uncle Darren, the one who saved me when I rode my bike down the steps when I was a little girl, assaulted me at my grandmother's house one day when I was taking care of his kids. Apparently unstable, he came in yelling at me as if I were my father. "Round one, let's see what you can do, kid. Round two, round three." Every time I'd get up, he'd beat me down again or hit me by my crotch.

I finally managed to pick up a tray to try to block him, but he still was able to beat me in the face. Finally, he pulled me up by my hair and the back of my shirt and dragged me toward the kitchen. He was going for a knife and said he was going to end it for me. As he was backing me toward a window with the intention of putting me through it, I blacked out. When I came to, he was kicking me in the face. Finally, my grandmother ran into the house—my cousin had run to get her—and it ended.

At the hospital, it was determined that he bruised my kidneys when he kicked me in the stomach, a part I didn't even remember.

I felt ashamed, the way victims do, as if it's somehow their fault. The episode really threw my energy off. I felt very uneven, and vulnerable, in a way that I never had been. At the same time, the incident heightened any sense I already had that the world is a place where you have to have your game face on, be a fighter.

Darren never tried to apologize. Soon after the attack, I gained a lot of weight and was up to 270 once more. Then, I guess to try to "erase" the incident, I pretty quickly lost 80 pounds with the help of an over-the-counter weight-loss product.

I wasn't thin but I was "in range." I started going to New York

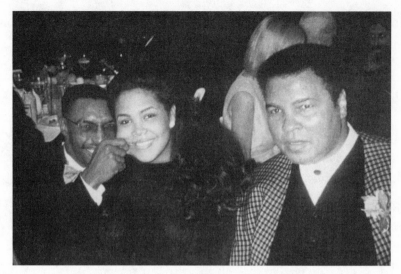

MY BROTHER, MUHAMMAD JR., AND ME AT MY SISTER RASHEEDA'S WEDDING.
(OUR FATHER IS CLEARLY SOMEWHERE ELSE AT THIS MOMENT!)
I WAS TWENTY-ONE OR TWENTY-TWO.

more. I was meeting more people and was feeling more and more that something would click. It soon did. I was approached by an immensely powerful woman in fashion named Catherine Lippincott—I was in my early twenties at this point—and she invited me to be an advisory board member of Lane Bryant.

I flew to a Lane Bryant show in New York directly from a meeting with my father in Dallas, where I had been interviewing him for a story I was pulling together for a special *Woman's Day* publication on famous sports figures and their take on women in sports. I remember there were tornadoes in Texas as I was driving to the airport—the flight started out extremely turbulent—and the Chaka Khan song "Through the Fire" was playing on the radio, mirroring in its words my fear mixed with anticipation.

On the face of it, it's a love song, but it's also a song about a new beginning that's too good to say "no" to, even though making the shift will be difficult . . .

I know you're afraid of what you feel
You still need time to heal . . .

The lyrics then urge you to go after your dream, "through the fire," if necessary, implying that what lies ahead will prove incredible almost beyond what you can imagine.

Storms forced us to land in New York behind schedule, and I had to rush from the airport over to Lane Bryant. But as anxious as I was about being late, I remember very distinctly that the taxi radio was playing the exact same song. It felt like, from outside of me, something was getting connected to something else.

Still, because the flight had been late, I was totally discombobulated once I arrived. I dropped my bag and some papers all over the floor. As I bent over to pick them up, from behind me a voice said, "My God, if your face looks as good as your ass . . . turn around so I can see you."

It was Mary Duffy, who worked for Eileen Ford. She brought me to the Ford Modeling Agency, where I met Eileen's son, Bill, and then Eileen Ford herself. Eileen was extremely complimentary, saying I was very beautiful, very all-American, with a clean, natural look, something that came from the inside out. She also said I had the "it" factor—a certain energy, or presence. I couldn't believe it was me she was talking about, but I lapped it all up. Soon afterward, I was signed—as a plus-size model—and there it was. I no longer was simply fat. I was fat *professionally*.

4

CRISIS POINT

never did end up modeling. I'd show up for a shoot, or go out on a call with other models to see if I'd get chosen, and then refuse to follow through. I didn't want to model a bra. "I don't do mini-skirts," I'd say. "I don't do sexy clothes." Lane Bryant's wanting me to wear fishnets and a fuchsia top was just not okay.

But there was also more to it. I was gaining back the eighty pounds I had lost. Even by the time Ford took my glossy photo to send around, my weight was up over two hundred pounds. The over-the-counter product I had been using was a quick fix, and nothing more. My weight was coming back to haunt me.

Still, on some level I was starting to become the person I needed to be to have my band surgery. In fact, while the operation didn't take place until August 6, 2004, my inner preparation began five and

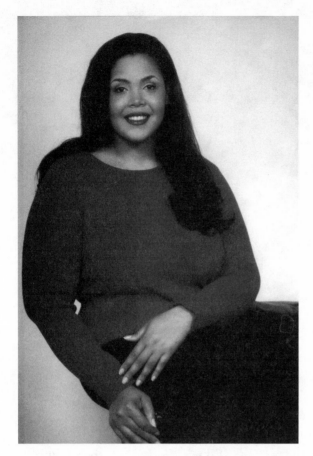

a half years earlier, on January 21, 1999, when I hadn't been with Ford all that long. That was the day my son, Jacob, was born.

It's almost as though I could draw a line between those two dates. But not a smooth one. It was, in fact, a tortured path, and the very darkest time of my life in many ways.

Jacob himself was such a *huge* source of light and happiness, my greatest blessing ever. But he was my candle in a tunnel. The light he shed made me know just how dark things really were and became the true motivation to make my life better. I had to change my standards for myself because I wanted to become a better person for my son. I

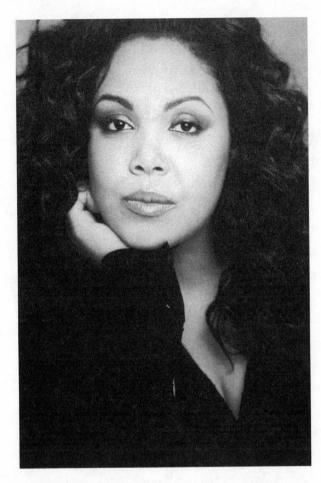

MY FIRST OFFICIAL FORD
MODEL PHOTO. YOU CAN
SEE I HAD ALREADY
GAINED BACK WEIGHT
SINCE THE TEST SHOOT.
Courtesy Ford Models, Inc.

had always had an ambitious streak, but my expectations were, for the first time, truly elevated. It wasn't just about covering my bases financially anymore.

Yet while I knew from the day Jacob was born that I somehow had to do more for myself, be better, knowing and achieving are two different things.

I guess you could say this period of my life, the last part of the winding journey toward accomplishing what I needed to do, actually began a year and a half before Jacob's birth, when I was twenty-three.

A friend of mine told me there was a man she thought I should meet—but I shooed her off. Still a virgin and insecure about my body, I had done very little dating and, while interested, just didn't think I had it in me to be with a man, or really be wanted by one.

Soon after, however, I went to a play in Philadelphia about the fighter Jack Johnson. During intermission, Joe Frazier's daughter, Jacqui, with whom I'm very close friends despite our fathers' boxing-ring antagonism and despite her own in-the-ring bouts with my sister Laila, said she wanted me to meet someone. His name was Spencer.

I remember shaking his hand, and our eyes kind of locked. A friend who was with me sensed it. Everyone sensed it. For the first time in my life, I walked away with feelings that other girls must have by the time they're in their teens but which must have been lying dormant in me.

At the end of the play, Spencer bought a six-foot sketch of Jack Johnson. I told him, sticking a toe into the bracing waters of flirting, that I wanted it. He responded, "I guess you'll have to come to my farm now." I said, "Okay," but that was the end of it—or so I thought.

A few months later, I went to see the Philadelphia Dance Company with the friend who originally said she wanted to set me up with someone. She walked me over to a man and said, "This is the guy I wanted you to meet." It was Spencer.

Soon after, I went to visit Spencer on his farm, and we started dating. At that point I weighed under 225 and did everything I could not to gain any more. It was a period of intense dieting. I budgeted my calories as tightly as possible, eating very little and going hungry, just to maintain. I'd work out on a treadmill, walk everywhere. I thought about liposuction.

Fortunately, my weight didn't seem to bother Spencer. He kept

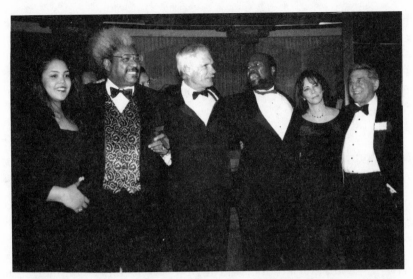

A MORE UNLIKELY CAST OF CHARACTERS YOU COULDN'T DREAM UP: ME (AGE 23), DON KING, TED TURNER, CONGRESS OF RACIAL EQUALITY NATIONAL CHAIRMAN ROY INNIS, MARCIA CLARK, AND OPERA SINGER ROBERT MERRILL AT CORE'S 1998 MARTIN LUTHER KING JR., FEDERAL HOLIDAY CELEBRATION. Courtesy Congress of Racial Equality/Tom Casino.

dating me even though I was considerably bigger than he was. That allowed us to move our relationship to another level, and the rest, as they say, is history.

During my pregnancy I met Jane Pauley again. It was at an awards ceremony for women in television. I didn't know yet that I was pregnant, but I already was feeling different. I had walked eighty blocks up to Lincoln Center on New York's West Side—my usual calorie-burning kind of thing—and was kind of out of it. I had fallen in a mud puddle and then realized I had lost my wallet and couldn't take a cab, so I arrived dirty and sweaty.

I was there as a presenter and remember thinking, "Damn, she's watching." But she was wonderful. She remembered me, and was so gracious.

As for Spencer and me, to this day we love each other, and we both do whatever it takes to make the best life for our son. Also, he has always stuck by me, to our friendship, and has seen to it as best as he could that I was successful in whatever ways I wanted to be. But we never married.

So when Jacob was born, I felt I needed to provide for my son. It's not that Spencer has ever denied or ever would deny Jacob or me a thing. There is always that cushion. But because of my own childhood, during which my father was often not there for me and my mother was left vulnerable, it was crucial to me to create security for my son and myself. The moment I looked into my son's eyes, I said, "You're going to get better than I had—the security, the stability."

That's why, nine days after Jacob was born, I was out working, hawking computer products through a very lucrative contract I had managed to sign with a company specializing in education software. It was on-the-road work—I logged more than a hundred thousand

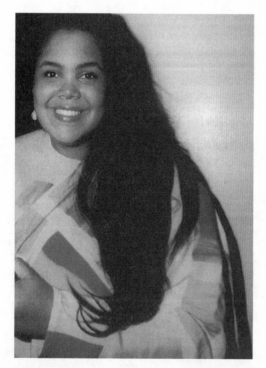

I'M ABOUT TWENTY-FIVE IN THIS SHOT, AND I WEIGH ABOUT 310 POUNDS.

frequent-flyer miles that year—so I was feeding myself in hotel rooms across America. And I *ate*—and ate and ate.

By the time Jacob was a year old, I was up to 325 pounds, by far the highest weight I had ever been at in my life.

It wasn't just being a new mother, and it wasn't just working at a fast pace in a high-stress job, and it wasn't just living out of hotel minibars and ordering in from restaurants. There were other things that had gone on that had really shaken me.

One was that my great-grandmother Reba, the seamstress, died the day I found out I was pregnant. But as painful as that was—no one I was close to had died before then—it was nothing like the deaths of two teenage boys who had always been virtual cousins to me. Our mothers had been friends forever.

Brian was sixteen, and Darnell was fourteen. They died in a car accident the day after Christmas, when I was well into my ninth month.

Those two boys had been angels all through my pregnancy, keeping me company and making me feel great. But looking back, I see there had also been something eerie in it. Brian kept saying he was going to be the baby's godfather, repeatedly insisting on it even though I had already told him that was fine with me.

And Darnell had spoken of his death all the previous summer. He said he would die of a brain tumor someday.

When the coroner's report was released, it said Darnell died of massive brain injuries—close enough to his prediction to send chills up my spine.

Then Jacob came almost three weeks late—on what would have been Brian's seventeenth birthday. The connection to the idea of someone being a godfather, being close to God for a child's sake, was so palpable. Although I had always prayed, I felt like that's when I really knew God existed.

At the same time, however, the way events had lined up created a lot of panic and anxiety. My introduction to motherhood was shadowed by the fact that a woman I had known my whole life had lost both her children. The birth was spliced together with tragedy. Of course, always looming in the back of my mind was that my parents were sick almost as far back as I could remember—my father with his Parkinson's and my mother with lupus—so parents and children losing each other was *always* something I had worried about.

At the beginning, when Jacob had just been born, I was overwhelmed that God had given me this person, and the moments of panic were intermittent. But as time went on, I got worse, paranoid about losing my son. That's why I always took Jacob around the country with me. I could have handed him off to a nanny—Spencer would have taken care of that, and by that point, perhaps, I could have gone directly to my father—but I didn't trust anyone else to take care of him. I had so much fear of being separated from him and having something happen to him. I lived in fear that whole first year. It was parasitic, eating away at the core of me even as I was stuffing myself.

My way of coping, besides eating, was to overcompensate. All first-time parents walk around with a certain level of worry for their child's safety and well-being, but I was the mother who was checking for SIDS constantly. I was the one who was always checking that the car seat was hooked up right. At the same time, I'd always be asking myself questions like "Is his environment clean enough?" His clothes always had to be neatly put away. I was trying so hard to do everything right to the point that I wasn't paying any attention whatsoever to myself.

In that state—survival mode—day after day, deeper and deeper, I was losing myself. It was like a drowning sensation. I denied myself everything—except food. Eating was the valve I'd use to try to let some of the panic escape.

I'd order room service—elaborate dinners late at night. There were also things like hoagies, sandwiches with chips. I'd eat a thousand calories' worth of food and try to fool myself by washing it down with Diet Coke.

On the rare nights that Jacob and I were home, I developed a very bad habit of eating bowls of cereal just before going to bed. I'd tell myself it was okay because the cereal was healthy. Then I couldn't fall asleep and would go back downstairs and get another bowl. Still, the hunger would kick in again before I was able to nod off. I'd go make a grilled cheese sandwich.

While out on the road, I thought nothing of eating thirty, forty pieces of sushi at a sitting. Again, it was "okay," I told myself, because sushi was a "healthy" food.

Ironically, during my pregnancy I had gained only fourteen pounds, while my mother had gained forty! We would do Indian food buffets—saag paneer, samosas, basmati rice. But I hadn't hungered for the food. It was more about keeping company. Yet here I was a year after Jacob's birth, a hundred pounds heavier than when he was born.

When you wake up one day and find yourself at 325 pounds, you don't have a relationship with yourself, much less anyone else. I was running on a treadmill, yet in a fog. Instead of acting in life, I was reacting—the very thing I didn't want to be doing. I wasn't taking charge, and my emotional chaos was playing itself out on my body.

At one point during my heaviest weight, I ran into my father at a fund-raiser hosted at Ethel Kennedy's house. He turned a corner—neither of us had been aware that the other was there—and just looked at me. The only thing I could read from his eyes was sadness. He was happy to see me, but concerned. He knew from the way I looked that I had lost my balance.

He was right, of course, and my shame and loss of dignity kept being revisited upon me in all kinds of ways that thin, or even moderately fat people, never even have to think about, let alone experience.

I had entered a whole new world of being overweight that became part and parcel of every moment of my waking life. There was no more escaping awareness about my body, even momentarily.

I remember getting on an airplane once with Jacob and pulling the seat belt as far as it would go but not being able to close it. Too mortified to ask for an extender, I took the seat belt and just kind of tucked it underneath my top on both sides to make it look like I was safely fastened in. I was willing to risk my well-being to avoid drawing further attention to my size.

Another time, I had just come in the back door of my house and was sitting in a wooden kitchen chair when a friend and some neighborhood kids came by, and right in front of them, the chair burst under me. Lying on the floor, I kept trying to cover my legs so no one would see how big they were. It wasn't until the next day that I saw I had a massive leg bruise. The embarrassment of having done in the chair and ending up on the floor was stronger than my body's own pain signals.

A while after Jacob was born, I ended up with a urinary tract infection that led to sepsis, and I had to be hospitalized. My health situation was grave, but all I could think about was having to walk from my room in a hospital gown, my arms and some of my legs exposed, to get blood work and other tests. I could barely keep the thing wrapped around my behind.

There were day-to-day things, too. I would have to rock myself out of bed because my feet swelled and my knees ached and my back hurt; I couldn't move like other people. I also had to rock and then squeeze myself out of a car. People would look—disgust or pity on their faces, or sometimes just unabashed stares, the way people dumbly watch a car wreck.

You never think to yourself at those moments that others have no right to be entertained by you as a freak show, that you're nobody else's business. You just feel the heat rise to your face. You wish you could disappear, and that makes it all the harder to get a handle on yourself. How can you begin to think for yourself when the whole world is constantly weighing in, either placing blame or otherwise putting in their two cents, even without words? You can't keep private that which is most private about you.

And so while I had told myself when Jacob was born that things were going to be better, I wasn't even able to find a way to cope, never taking time to settle or evaluate, so to speak. I hadn't had an easy time of it in the past; there was always some kind of family dynamic at work or some crisis that made focusing on my weight too difficult. Now my weight *was* the crisis. How could I tend to my inner life when my most *visible* problem had overtaken all other concerns?

Still, even with all the emotional handicapping that comes with being obese, I tried to find a way to keep from overeating—through diet pills.

I started with the prescription pill Tenuate, then would switch back and forth with Hydroxycut, which is over-the-counter. At the same time, my mother moved across the country to California for a year, which helped because we had become codependent on each other when it came to eating.

I ended up losing close to a hundred pounds, pretty much right back to where I had started.

But—and this was very scary to me—the diet pills wouldn't work after a while. The hunger returned. Or I needed to get off them because of side effects—I'd start bruising easily. Or I'd get overconfident, thinking I had the problem licked, under my thumb. So I'd go off the pills and gain back thirty, forty, fifty pounds, and get terrified. Then the cycle would start all over again.

I'd lose twenty pounds and feel ecstatic about it—"I'm the greatest person in the world"—then, two weeks later, gain it all back and feel depressed. "What's wrong with me? I'm horrible." It was very yo-yo.

The number on the scale that particularly haunted me was 220. I couldn't get below that, and it was scary because my father's fighting weight had been 219. It played into my psyche that I couldn't get below the weight of this man—my own flesh and blood—who was six feet, four inches.

Confusing the issue was the fact that people in certain circles kept telling me I looked good. "You're okay, Khaliah." I'd keep hearing it from agents and publicists, which made sense since I *had* signed on as a plus-size model. I was *supposed* to be big. Also, out of nowhere, or perhaps just noticed by me for the first time, there was no shortage of interest from men. Some, I suppose, wanted a piece of my celebrity status as my father's daughter, but others genuinely liked my shape. Certain men really do prefer women with a lot of weight on them.

Still, inside myself, I knew my body wasn't where I needed it to be. I didn't like my joints aching, always feeling winded, wearing through shoes quickly. (Take a look at a very fat person's feet. They're as distorted as the rest of an obese body.)

Paralleling this disconnect between what people were telling me and how I felt about myself both mentally and physically were some interesting, even fruitful, turns that my life was taking.

While Bill Ford should have been furious with me for refusing to do photo shoots, he never gave up on me, not even when my weight climbed to more than three hundred—too plus even for plus-size modeling. Instead, he used his contacts to help me develop my own line of clothing for women on the Home Shopping Network, including plus-size clothing that I knew big women would be comfortable wearing. I was thrilled because as a plus-size woman myself, I never liked the styles I found on the racks. They fell short of what I needed to feel okay. I wanted to offer clothes that would flatter larger women and make the clothes affordable at the same time.

The line was very successful, which I think had to do with its focus on diversity of all kinds. For one thing, the clothing celebrated the diversity of women's bodies, even the diversity of a woman's body within a single month. I used elastic rather than buttons to camouflage the monthly ups and downs, but I hid the stretchability. No one would ever know elastic was in the clothing, and that allowed women not to have to spend extra money on two sets of clothing for their "good" and "bad" weight days.

I also went for diversity in a woman's lifestyle—a black jacket, for instance, that she could wear with jeans but that she could also dress up with rhinestones and wear to a cocktail party. It gave different pieces of clothing more than one use, so a woman could buy something she felt great about and not feel guilty spending on it.

Finally, it was very important to me to celebrate ethnic and cultural diversity. A work suit might have a mandarin collar and frog toggles with a quarter-inch split in the cuff, giving a woman an educated, artsy look yet with a hint of Asian influence. Or I might do a plain white T-shirt with a little Peruvian art at the bottom—subtle, not overwhelming. I always offered simple, basic coordinates, too—a skirt in solid colors, for instance, so that you could pull in some ethnic influence if you wanted to add flair, or keep it all plain to go in for a job interview.

On the heels of doing the clothing line, I became involved with plus sizes for Simplicity, a company that creates sewing patterns for women who make their own clothes. I don't design the patterns myself, but I work with a designer to whom I give creative input. "I don't think linen's right here. I think it should be in crepe; turquoise, not pale blue, would be right here; I think this is two inches too small in the behind," and so on. You can buy the patterns in Wal-Mart, Kmart, and Joanna's Fabrics.

The clothing endeavor has been and continues to be successful, which has both calmed me and helped with my self-esteem.

I was also pleased during those years to continue doing a fair amount of charity work, which helped me feel connected to my father.

My father, all his bluster and bravado to the contrary, is extraordinarily humble. He takes nothing and no one for granted, and it was always his expectation that I would follow his example.

In fact, if you are with my father and deny someone in need, fear for your life. He has taken his shoes off in the street and given them to someone without.

My charity work was both formal and informal. Formally, I was involved with a number of organizations. One was the Special Olympics; I had a hand in getting my father and other athletes to donate sports memorabilia to raise funds. I also did fund-raising for Big Brothers Big Sisters, and worked at the local level to get computers donated to schools.

I lectured, too, talking to school-age children about HIV and to college students about the benefits of embracing ethnic and cultural diversity.

Informally, I tried to follow in my father's footsteps by not turning a blind eye when I saw people in need. Once, after leaving Jacob off at Spencer's house, I came upon a woman who was basically living out of a shopping cart. She wouldn't accept my offer of help, but I managed to at least get her to take a blanket and a couple of pillows that I brought her from home.

At another point, when I was living in Center City, Philadelphia, where homelessness was rampant, I would encounter women with children and bring them food, or give them cab fare to get somewhere, or stuff some money into their hands, or make some phone calls to see about getting them some help.

I knew all of this was right. I was glad to be able to reach out to others. But even though I hadn't lost my heart, and even though I had found business success through the fashion lines, I still wasn't able to reach out to *myself.* In fact, trying to get everything just right was keeping me from myself.

A lot of overweight women find themselves in this predicament. They're very accomplished, perfectionists even, and they're terrific about extending themselves to others. But the one thing they can't do is lose weight. And their anxiety around that only fuels the problem. They keep doing more and more, and become harder and harder on themselves, to compensate for the one area in their lives in which they haven't had success. And all it does is take them even further away from being able to do anything about their weight in a pragmatic way because they're so busy focusing their energies elsewhere. Which, in turn, only makes them beat themselves up more: "I can do everything else. Why won't my body do *this*?" The upshot: to deal with the frustration they do the very thing that's contributing to so much of their unhappiness. They eat, and the whole cycle then ratchets itself up another notch. I was definitely one of those women.

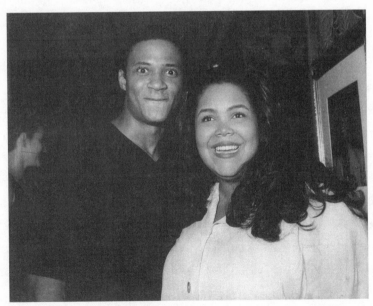

THE ACTOR HERE PORTRAYED MY FATHER IN A PLAY. I WAS IN MY MID-TWENTIES.

At the same time, I was looking backward at my life and living as a victim, not accepting responsibility for my weight, rather than reaching forward to find solutions. "I had a difficult childhood. I wouldn't be so fat if I hadn't lost so much of my youth"; "Spencer and I would be together if I were thinner" (which was not true—Spencer found me desirable no matter what my weight, and our breakup had nothing to do with that); "my weight is keeping me from being attractive to other men"; "if this hadn't happened and that hadn't happened, I wouldn't be so disgusting." In other words, I was trying to justify my feeling that life was happening to me rather than something I could direct. It was a toxic mental formula, because while you can rightly hold the people in your past accountable, only you, in the present, can be responsible for what happens going forward.

Unfortunately, all of that refusing to be responsible for myself was only fueling the hunger—both physically and spiritually. Because I was feeding myself platitudes rather than truths. And that, in turn, led to more overeating to shove down the truths, so to speak.

Nothing was relieving the spiritual hunger, and the only thing that ever relieved the physical hunger was the diet pills. But you can't take diet pills to make you feel not hungry your whole life. And not just because they stop working after a while or because of the relatively minor side effects they gave me. I found out that some diet pills can affect your heart. I had heard a story about a friend's mother who died suddenly in her kitchen from having taken diet pills years before. They had ruined her heart valves. That terrified me, especially because I was getting chest pains—probably from panic, but it made my level of fear spiral upward. You know how your head can play games with you.

It was getting to the point that even as I kept eating, all I could think about was my weight. I logged countless hours on obesity-health.com. I even thought about getting gastric bypass surgery, the kind Carnie Wilson had. I went very far in the process, having the doctors send me the presurgical kit. But I couldn't go through with it.

For one thing, I knew that for all practical purposes, it wasn't reversible, and that scared me. Also, I knew that people who had the surgery couldn't ever eat normally again. You had to take tiny bites and chew so well that certain foods became tasteless liquids or "cotton balls" in your mouth. And you had to virtually give up certain foods, like sweets, because they could cause the "dumping syndrome"—the sweats, faintness, nausea, vomiting, and diarrhea. Then, too, I felt that if I went for the surgery, I was defeated, that after a lifetime of doing battle with my body, my body would have won and the operation would be the treaty of defeat I'd have to live with for the rest of my life.

But the biggest fear, bigger than any emotional reservations, was the fear of dying. I was well acquainted with the statistic that as many as one in twenty-five patients suffer—and sometimes die from—problems such as intestinal fluid leakage into the abdominal cavity following the operation. And I had heard about other life-threatening complications—blood clots that make their way to the lungs, heart attacks, respiratory failure.

I couldn't take those chances. I couldn't risk having a leak or some other uncontrollable complication and leaving my child. I wanted to live for my son.

Yet at the same time I felt I was going to die from the weight—literally. So I was frozen. I couldn't move forward, and I couldn't move backward, and I couldn't even move within the present. And frozen like that, I was dying slowly; my spirit was dying. More than five years had gone by since Jacob's birth, I was turning thirty, and in some ways I felt like I was already dead, that I had succumbed to something.

It was more than that I had kissed away my twenties and was miserable. It was more, much more, than that I couldn't be naked with anybody, couldn't wear a backless dress, couldn't go to the beach—all the things a person should be able to do.

It was raw pain for me even to have a photograph taken. How many times did I run from a video camera or purposely cut myself out of a group so that I couldn't be seen through a lens? I was trying, literally, not to exist, to leave no record of myself. I had taken myself out of the game. I would think to myself, "If I die tomorrow, what photos of me would my son have?"

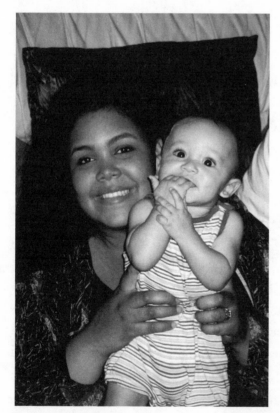

JACOB WASN'T EVEN A YEAR OLD YET, AND ALREADY I WAS AS HEAVY AS I COULD BE AT 325 POUNDS.

Thankfully, I had a friend who read all this in me. Wiggy—really Arlene Olson—is someone I met through a public relations effort for the Salvation Army. We became very close. Even she and my son bonded in such a strong way.

Wiggy was spearheading a project in which people overcoming addiction to drugs or other struggles and who needed job skills received training in the culinary arts through a catering program called Soup's On!, which put her on the rehabilitative end of overcoming an addiction or other hard knocks. I was brought in to be a face on the effort, which is how we got to know each other. But over time, Wiggy saw me becoming less confident, holding back. She'd see me wearing the same outfit again and again. She'd see me wearing tons of black. She'd see me shying away from the camera.

She was concerned for me because when we first met, I had seemed really resilient, with a lot of energy, even with all the physical problems my weight caused me. So she knew it was more than just a fat person being embarrassed about her weight. She knew it was more than someone just yo-yoing up and down, that the struggle had gone beyond pounds toward serious depression, but that the weight was very much tied into my emotional state.

Finally, one day she turned to me and said, "Khaliah, you just need to go for it."

"What are you talking about?" I asked.

"I have a cousin in New York who got this thing, a surgery for weight loss."

"No, I can't have the surgery," I said.

"It's not the usual one," Wiggy insisted. She had to hold up her hand so I would let her finish. "They put a band around your stomach. My cousin already lost seventy-something pounds, and she can still eat. She can even *adjust* the band. We've eaten out together. She's able to enjoy food. Go to the Web site. Read what the two surgeons have to say. It's a team. Fielding and Ren."

I resisted. I couldn't bear the thought of surgery. All I could think about was Jacob, about the possibility of not being here for him. But in a way, I already wasn't here.

So I went to the Web site and read an essay by Fielding, one of the two surgeons. He had this stomach band surgery himself. He had had a fat childhood, a difficult young adulthood. He, too, had overcompensated through overachieving. He "lost seventy pounds four times."

He talked about "the pain and humiliation of always being huge and fighting it" and spoke of how "it just exhausted" him. He talked about his presurgery days, "wanting a life," about how he had always tried to have one even though many think fat people don't make an effort. He said, "Try being two hundred pounds, then being three hundred pounds."

I *knew* this person. And he knew me, even though we had never met.

At first I just sat there. Then I cried. Then I laughed. Then I went and prayed and thanked God. I was going to be able to save myself.

DR. FIELDING'S STORY

Here is an abridged and slightly edited version of the essay by Dr. Fielding that I found on the Internet before going to see him. He calls it "Everybody Dreams." For the complete essay, go to http://thinforlife.med.nyu.edu/news/stories

Everybody dreams. What do obese people dream about? Sex, of course, everyday fears, weird things, just like everyone else.

Above all else, though, they dream about being thin, free of hunger, and looking normal.

They want a life, to be healthy, to come off multiple medications, to live longer, to be alive for their families, to play with their children. They want to get a job, get a promotion, have sex, get pregnant, have a child, sleep without a C-PAP mask, have their wife sleep in the same room because the snoring has stopped! You know, a normal life. Stuff like sitting in a movie seat, a plane seat, on a toilet seat, a bus seat. Not to mention walk up five stairs, up the street, out of the house, anywhere, without gasping. . . . Go to the beach, the gym, a clothing store without feeling like a freak show. Stuff like being the one who moves during sex, actually seeing their own penis or vulva.

How do I know all this? Easy. In the last eleven years, I have operated on more than four thousand morbidly obese patients, and I've heard it all four thousand times. They just want a life. Sure, they're scared. It's a big step. But hell, nothing else has worked.

Most have been to Jenny Craig and Weight Watchers at least three times, taken all the pills, done all the diets, sensible or not, done the walking, the gym, the nutritionists, the calorie counting, and the starving. None of it has worked long-term. So they come in, nervous, a deep part of them sure it's a con like everything else, ready for failure, yet desperate for success.

How else do I know? Easy—I'm one of my patients. I've had the surgery, too. It's weird hearing four thousand people tell you your own life story.

Growing up in Australia, I was the fat kid in elementary school. I saw my first doctor to see if I had an endocrine gland problem when I was ten. I didn't—I just ate too much. So, I was put on my first diet. It was torture. I cheated all the time because I was starving. I was very active, played all the sports, and was also quite brainy. We never had a TV, so I read a lot and played music. I just ate all the time. Clothes were a problem. Nothing fit, so Mom made them. I was called every simile and metaphor for fat imaginable. Not surprisingly, I became completely determined to beat all the bastards. I lived starving hungry.

When I was nearly fifteen certain aspects of my life started to change. A teacher, Brian Short, taught that pursuit of excellence was a good thing and that winning was good. My father taught me that all people have equal rights. So armed with a fierce will to win and a brain, I set out to conquer the world—and have done so pretty much.

I have a beautiful partner and four great kids. I became a surgeon by age twenty-nine and was in private practice by age thirty-four. I played rugby quite well and later coached, and I played two musical instruments well enough to be in a band until I was forty-three. I read thousands of books, listened to masses of music, traveled the world, surfed at the beach, bought a share in a house in Burgundy, and drank more wine than was strictly necessary. I simply took life by the throat.

I find surgery a joy. I have operated as a surgeon in Britain, France, Japan, Singapore, Hong Kong, Bangkok, and the United States. I love teaching, surely appear arrogant to many, and make minimally invasive surgery look as hard as pulling on socks.

All this, yet I just could not stop eating. I could never control hunger. The pain and humiliation of always being hungry and fighting it just exhausted me. Despite living a life where false modesty would have been a wasted emotion, deep down I felt like a failure.

Pick a vegetable—done 'em all. I have been on a soup-and-broccoli diet, grapefruit, Israeli army, Pritikin, high carb, low carb, high protein, no protein, starvation, eat what you like, run eight miles a day, do weights till my shirts bust, swim a mile a day and die of boredom. How about pills? Done them all, too—Adifax, Phentermine, Optifast, Zoloft. I was always hungry.

Since 1980, I have lost seventy pounds four times. Each time took about eighteen months. I felt like a different person with each go-round. I'm strong, confident, aggressive, very sexual, and in control. Then, *whoosh—blink,* and it's all back on, plus some.

It never goes away. Try being two hundred pounds, then being three hundred pounds. You still think like a two-hundred-pound tough guy, but you look and feel like a big, smart, aggressive blimp. Imagine Pussy, not Tony Soprano. Therefore, you start back on the road, dieting, running, working too hard, overcompensating in everything to override how awful you feel.

That was the cycle of my life for twenty years. Watching the Broadway version of *The Full Monty,* when the fat guy sang a gentle love song—"You Rule My World"—not to his wife lying next to him in bed but to his stomach, to his hunger, I sat in the theater crying.

Then I got sick—all kinds of sick. Asthma, reflux, sleep apnea, depression, and finally heart arrhythmias. I was in my forties, taking ten medications a day, in the middle of a midlife crisis to end them all.

Working like a lunatic, out of breath all the time, tired all the time.

As well as my usual surgery for various health problems, I was doing ten bariatric operations a week. I had been converted to the cause four years previously and was very happy with the results. Strangely enough, this was the most satisfying work I had done—making people healthy and happy, giving them a normal life. The patients' stories were all the same as mine.

Still, I held off and held off. One day I cracked. After staring in the mirror and *really* looking at the protruding stomach, the round face, and the discouraged look in my eyes, I weighed myself—and nearly fainted at the figure: 310 pounds. I sat down, rang my friend in Melbourne, Paul O'Brien, and booked myself for a banding procedure.

Many doctors have written about being on the other side, on the receiving end. We all find it an awkward place. As a group, surgeons are famed for their inability to give in, to admit frailty. Flying to Melbourne to have the surgery, I was scared, nervous about powerlessness, anxious about complications. Yet I knew it was less risky to have weight-loss surgery than to remain obese. And I was thrilled to finally be gaining control. I had seen it help so many of my patients. I would gain control.

I have. Within a week of the operation, my excess weight began to melt away. Even more startling, I had no hunger pangs. Before surgery, I was forever hungry; hunger always won, which is why I kept regaining weight after I had lost it. But now, that brutal force that had driven me off so many rigid diets in the past no longer hounded me.

Seven years later, no hunger, and ninety-five pounds down. I feel great, am off all of my pills, have boundless energy to do anything I want without getting tired. All it took was one night in the hospital, three days off work, five tiny incisions. Eating slowly, eating small meals, never being hungry. That's the biggest blessing, never being hungry.

Who'd believe that such a simple thing as a band, a little piece of silicone with an internal adjustable balloon, could render such a service? Hunger no longer rules my world. A fat boy's dream has come true. I still dream about sex, too, but I don't get out of breath, even in my dreams.

5

GUT-LEVEL BOND

I could feel my stomach clenching into knots as the elevator climbed to the tenth floor. The whole drive up from Philadelphia to the New York University Medical Center in Manhattan, I was nervous, but now, after years of thinking about obesity surgery yet putting it off, I was finally here for my pre-op consult and felt out-and-out terrified. I wasn't at all sure that I could go through with it. The cold, clinical atmosphere of the hospital, the pained, worried looks of family members coming to see loved ones, the officialness of it all—it really ratcheted up my fear.

The trepidation dissipated when Dr. Fielding came over and introduced himself; I was now doing what I had set out to do rather than anticipating it, which always helps to quell anxiety. But in the place vacated by fear came grief, or maybe grief mixed with catharsis, I'm not sure. I grabbed my chest and welled up with tears.

Dr. Fielding didn't shake my hand. He put his arm around me and led me into his tiny consulting room, where we had, in certain ways, the most intimate conversation I've ever had. He was requiring me, in essence, to convince him that I was ready for the operation, which is to say I had to talk about myself and how I had come to be so heavy and had spent so much of my life fighting my weight. Then he opened up and shared with me some of his own experience, which, of course, is different in person from when you're reading it by yourself on the Internet.

From there, Dr. Fielding had my trust in him as a person, but I was still nervous about the surgery. I asked him if my stomach could rip. He said no, and lifted his shirt to let me feel his own abdomen so I could get a sense of the little boxlike reservoir placed in there with the band during the operation. From that little box, sort of like a flattened golf ball, water can be channeled to the band to tighten it and thereby decrease hunger (think of the band as a tiny life preserver filling up, going from deflated to taut around the upper part of the stomach).

I then asked him what my odds were of regaining any weight I lost. He said that I could regain lost weight if I wanted to, that there were ways to eat around the band. He added, however, that it's a very powerful tool that absolutely will allow you to remain thinner if you let it, and that it's not hard to cooperate with it.

Finally, I asked him if having a stomach band put in would shorten my life expectancy. I was most nervous for my five-year-old son. No, he answered. It wouldn't shorten my life expectancy; it would add to it.

Then he said, in a way surgeons don't usually say things, "Doll, don't wait." He explained to me that obesity is a disease, which a person could no better will away than heart disease or diabetes, and in almost all cases requires medical intervention because an obese body is hardwired for hunger in a way that a thin or moderately overweight body is not. That, in turn, enabled me to surrender.

Surrender has always been a hard concept for me to get my mind around. I don't think of myself as someone who gives up. But we talked about the fact that I wasn't surrendering my life, my spirit, the fight I had in me. I simply was surrendering the type of battle I had been waging against my weight and choosing a different plan of attack.

Admittedly, giving up a lifetime of serial dieting is no easy thing. As frustrating and defeating as it is, it's all you know. It's what you come to depend on to define your ups and downs, your own kind of equilibrium. Still, I had come too far by that point to turn back. I was, finally, willing to lie on a slab and let somebody cut into me for the purpose of freeing me from a struggle I had been having for as far back as I could remember.

Dr. Ren added to my resolve. I had seen her before on *Oprah* and met her briefly that day, and her straightforward, upbeat manner reeled me in. I wasn't put off by her beauty or size-two thinness, or even by the fact that she had never struggled with weight. I saw them as incentives. As always, I wanted to be that person who could walk into a room the way she did—confident, clearheaded, and with no messiness about her. It didn't hurt that, like me, she is of mixed-race heritage—both European and Asian. I felt that she, too, must have done her share of feeling like she belonged and didn't at the same time.

Driving home after the consult, I felt very excited. I couldn't believe I was finally going to have a chance to be thin. But for all Dr. Fielding's and Dr. Ren's reassurances, a part of me was still afraid I would die. Then I took a deep breath, let it out, and decided to allow myself be happy. There are times, and this was one of them, when you just have to insist on not going with your compulsion to drive yourself crazy.

From that point forward, I began to get excited with a type of feeling that I can only explain by way of saying it was like the feeling I had when I was pregnant. I was exhilarated, exhilarated about something happening inside me, a change growing within.

I then made what for me was a mistake—telling people about my plans. Some did support me unequivocally, including my mother. I also received unconditional support from two people I feel closer to than you can feel even with family members, brothers Joe and Jonny Abrams. I have talked about other friends who have been like family to me, but to give a sense of how bonded I feel with the Abrams brothers, it was Joe who managed to arrange a meeting between my father and me when I became pregnant so that I could tell him he was going to be a grandfather. I had been having difficulty reaching him, and Joe just kept chipping away at people in my father's entourage to clear a path for me.

Ironically, as close as we are, you might say I met Joe and Jonny through the Yellow Pages. When my mother was pregnant with my sister Lydia and needed a teeth cleaning before she gave birth, she chose a dental office out of the phone book, and the office manager assigned Joe to be her dentist. We had signs even then that there was a special connection. Lydia hadn't been moving much inside my mother, to the point that even her obstetrician was concerned. But whenever Joe came near, Lydia bounced around like crazy. After the birth, when my healthy younger sister came into the world, Joe gave my mother a baby gift.

Feelings remained close between the two families, but Joe and I ended up out of touch. It was around the time that I was trying to juggle college, trips to New York, and odd jobs to help keep my family afloat.

Then, when Lydia was already toddling around, somewhere between the age of one and two, I ran into Joe at four-thirty one morning at a Kinko's in King of Prussia, Pennsylvania. I was there pulling together a résumé and a bio for some spokesperson gig, and Joe was taking care of some of his office needs. We had each set our clocks to get up in the middle of the night to deal with unattended-to business.

There was an instant "recognition" between us; there's no other way to put it. And from then on our two families have been blended, even without any marriages between them. Joe has even filled in financial gaps that we weren't able to see our way through. And when his daughter, Jennifer, had her bat mitzvah, I lit one of the thirteen candles on her cake. Likewise, when my son was born, the Abramss were there to help celebrate the joy.

Strengthening our bond was that neither Joe nor Jonny was a stranger to struggles with weight. Jonny, in fact, grew to more than 400 pounds and was one of the very lucky few who managed to lose 225 of them via diet and exercise. He became not just thin but incredibly fit over a three-year period ending just before my surgery. The turning point for him had been that by a fluke, he missed being a passenger on one of the 9/11 flights. He was able to use his second chance to turn his life around in myriad ways.

It meant a particularly great deal that Jonny supported me in my decision, which was so different from how he solved his own weight problem. He was able to accept that we each go our own path.

But while Jonny and Joe and my mother rallied around me, others were more hesitant. Some, like my grandmother, were simply confused about how the surgery works. Others were concerned for my safety. Spencer, for instance, while supportive, was apprehensive.

Then there were the out-and-out doubters, various friends and colleagues who tried to frighten me out of going through with it. Comments ranged from the tame ("Come on, give Weight Watchers one more try") to the faintly patronizing ("You're a big, strong healthy girl, just accept yourself") to the truly damning ("I've heard people die getting that kind of thing, you're the mother of a young child").

That's when I realized it was a mistake for me to tell *anyone*. I ended up counting the yeas and nays, as if what I was going to do was predicated on the voting tally, and finally decided that I couldn't afford to hear any of it, positive or negative, just then. I was frightened enough on my own. I didn't need anyone else weighing in.

I had several weeks of keeping my own counsel, as it was a while before the actual surgery. In part that was because Drs. Fielding and Ren's practice is so busy, but also, there are certain people you have to see besides the surgeons who determine your readiness for the procedure, including a psychologist and a dietitian. The psychologist makes a formal determination about whether your head is in the right place (and evaluates people's expectations of what the surgery will do for them), and the dietitian talks to you about how your eating style is going to change so that you know what you're getting into. It's sort of like a test that the dietitian gives you, and you have to pass it to be cleared for the operation.

You also have to get blood tests, a urine analysis, an EKG, and a chest X-ray. The surgeons want a baseline of all kinds of things from those screenings, like your cholesterol level and blood sugar level, so they can have before-and-after measurements of these clinical aspects of your health. They also want to assess the state of your body in preparation for the operation.

Finally, for a couple of weeks before the surgery, you have to go on a liquid fast. They want you to lose a little weight to shrink your liver, which sits above your stomach, so that it's easier to get to where they need to get during the operation.

Ironically, before the fast began, I started planning very carefully for my nutritional future, eating healthful, well-rounded meals with salads at dinner and fruits for snacks between meals. I wanted to get this right.

I also ate as if I already had the band—slowly, methodically, *mindfully*. I was trying to take my body for a test run.

But when the actual fast started, I lasted exactly two days. I was extremely careful those first forty-eight hours, drinking things like wheatgrass juice and even making my own Popsicles. Then something snapped itself broken, and I ended up sneaking solids here and there. For instance, I was afraid I wouldn't be able to fit bagels down my throat anymore, so one morning I ate most of one. I also had a slice of pizza once, and a piece of chicken breast another time.

It wasn't like I was going hog wild. I still took in most of my calories via the liquid fast, and I *was* able to forgo many of my favorites: macaroni and cheese, pastries, Indian food, sushi. But to this day I don't know why I risked sabotaging myself like that with the solids I did eat. I was even participating in a meditation program recommended by Drs. Fielding and Ren, whereby you listen to a tape that talks about positive recovery, about being in the right place, about healing well. But I wasn't able to talk myself out of eating solids now and then. I was too scared about the future.

I didn't say anything to Dr. Fielding at the time. I figured I'd decide closer to the surgery date how to deal with it—tell him and risk not having the operation, or not tell him and risk I-didn't-know-what.

As the surgery date drew closer, I drove up to New York with some family and friends, Jonny Abrams included, for a meeting with Sri Chinmoy. A world-renowned spiritual guide, Sri Chinmoy gives what he calls "a lifting up the world with a oneness-heart" award to honor those he feels have lifted the world themselves through good acts. He has bestowed the honor on thousands of people over the years, including some very famous ones—Pope John Paul II, Nelson

Mandela, Mother Teresa, and performers like Susan Sarandon and Sting, among others. He chose me, in part, because of my involvement with a program called Culture Project, a New York City–based theater group that gives voice to disenfranchised and politically marginalized people by staging plays that call attention to their plight.

During the award ceremony, Sri Chinmoy literally lifts the person who has metaphorically lifted others. You have to be weighed before the lifting, which was mortifying for me as there were about two hundred people watching, although I did try to let go and just be in the moment.

After being weighed, you walk onto a platform, underneath which Sri Chinmoy sits in a chair and pushes straight up on one or two handles. For three or four seconds while he's lifting, he's fully supporting the weight of the person on the platform.

It's a strength that goes beyond physical. Sri Chinmoy is about five feet eight inches and weighs about 165 pounds (while my weight hovered around 300 at the time)—and was about seventy years old at the time of my own lifting! But that's the point. Sri Chinmoy believes people have an unlimited capacity within themselves, an inner strength that they can use as a source of power to transform things outwardly. He believes a person can transcend herself. That's what he's celebrating with the lifting.

I took it as a sign. Although Sri Chinmoy was honoring me for an inner strength he felt I had already demonstrated by doing good works, I felt it was prophetic that I was getting his award right before my surgery. It said to me that I would be able to handle something I had never before in my entire life mustered up the strength to overcome, that I'd find inner fortitude to effect outer changes.

During the ceremony, Sri Chinmoy meditated with me; there were flowers everywhere to make it all beautiful as well as calming. And after the lifting, he sang a song he'd prepared just for the event.

He then gave me a medal. I was overwhelmed. I had never received such an award in my life, and no one had ever acknowledged my public service before.

I delivered a short speech expressing gratitude, after which Sri Chinmoy took my hand and kissed me, ending the ceremony by saying, "May all your dreams come true."

The countdown to the operation then began in earnest. In the remaining days leading up to the procedure, I would sit once again for hours in front of obesityhealth.com, speculating about how I would eat, how I would exercise. I did a lot of fooling around with a pencil and paper, too. Imagine if I lose thirty pounds by this date, fifty pounds by that date, by Christmas. Speculating, daydreaming, I let myself go with it, although the surgeons did warn me that weight loss with a gastric band is not typically as fast as with gastric bypass.

Finally, it was the night before the surgery. I spent a lot of time praying and hugging and kissing my son. He didn't know what was about to happen, and I didn't want him to know. I was really scared again, letting my imagination run away with the most horrible thoughts. But deep in there I was still excited. What would life feel like, I wondered, across the divide? I was now only hours away from finding out.

BECOMING A CANDIDATE FOR GASTRIC BANDING

Like Khaliah, most people who end up opting for a gastric band have struggled with obesity and the off-and-on dieting that goes with it for their entire lives. That's as it should be. The great majority of doctors, including us, would agree that surgery is not the first step for weight loss. You first have to work solely with the traditional dieting tools: changes in eating habits and exercise.

In fact, patients who have not put forth effort with lifestyle alterations to try to get a handle on their weight tend to have the same results with surgery as they always had with dieting. The reason is that the band isn't magic; it's a tool. Granted, it relieves hunger like magic, but it just won't do what it's supposed to if you can't make a commitment to following a sensible eating plan and putting some physical activity into your life. (The activity doesn't have to be exercise per se, although it does have to involve some moving around.) It's for that reason that people who state a willingness to make healthful food choices and, in addition, are ready to start dealing with their emotions directly rather than resort to emotional eating, are considered better candidates than those who make clear that they do not wish to give up eating at, say, fast-food restaurants or do not wish to give up drinking or perhaps excessive drug use.

Every surgeon—or surgical center—has somewhat different criteria for accepting prospective weight-loss surgery candidates. But most follow the recommendations from the 1991 National Institutes of Health Consensus Development Conference Statement on the Surgical Treatment of Obesity, which says that the patient should be at least one hundred pounds overweight, or have a body mass index (BMI) of at least forty, or a BMI of at least thirty-five with two co-morbidities—conditions tied to their weight, such as heart disease, diabetes, severe sleep apnea, severe osteoarthritis, and depression. (See the chart on pages 102 and 103 to find your BMI.)

How do you choose a gastric banding surgeon or surgical practice? One good way is to get a recommendation from someone who has already had a successful banding operation. You can also ask your primary care physician. In addition, through the American Society for Bariatric Surgery, you can find a listing of Centers of Excellence—hospitals that meet certain criteria for obesity surgery, including having a staff that is prepared to manage morbidly obese patients with "care and understanding"; at least 125 bariatric surgeries a year; support groups for people who have undergone band surgery; and long-term patient follow-up. For listings of Centers of Excellence, surf to www.asbs.org and click on *Health Care Professionals.* From there, go to *Centers of Excellence,* and a map of the country will come up. Click on your state to find the Centers of Excellence in your locale, along with links to each one.

You can also search for surgeons who practice at Centers of Excellence by clicking on *Patients,* entering your zip code, and then clicking on both *Practicing Surgeon/Physician Members* and *Centers of Excellence.* Also, click on *LB* for "laparoscopic banding" so you get surgeons who perform that particular surgery. (The American College of Surgeons—www.facs.org—has a similar listing.)

Questions to get answers to, either online or by phone once you identify either a Center of Excellence or a certain surgeon who might be the right pick:

1. Do the bariatric surgeons in the practice perform the procedure laparoscopically, with a few tiny incisions, rather than by cutting into the abdomen with a large incision?

2. How many gastric bandings has the surgical practice (or the surgeon) you have in mind performed? (At least twenty-five per surgeon is okay. At least one hundred provides better "insurance.")

3. What is their complication rate, including fatality rate and reoperation rate for band slippage or other problems?

4. Does the surgeon/hospital work with a bariatric anesthesiologist, who is used to working with very heavy people?

5. What is the follow-up program like, including frequency of visits, support staff seen by patients (psychologist? dietitian?), and design of support group (monthly visits, online chats, and so on).

6. Who performs the band adjustments? The surgeon? A nurse or nurse practitioner? A physician's assistant?

The touchy-feely part is just as important as the technical part.

7. Do you get the sense that the surgeon will be there for the long haul, when you need to go in for periodic band adjustments and may need to talk? You may not get to talk to the surgeon directly, but how his or her staff treats you may be able to tell you a lot about the atmosphere there.

8. What about his or her bedside/desk-side manner? Is it easy to converse with the surgeon/staff? Will you feel comfortable discussing your weight-loss struggles and also your concerns going forward?

9. Has the surgeon spearheaded support groups—patients who talk with one another both before and after surgery? (A good sign is a surgeon encouraging you to attend a support group of people who have already had the surgery before you undergo the operation so you can get all your questions answered from *their* perspective as well as from the doctor's.)

10. Is there an insurance specialist on staff to help you work with your insurance carrier and submit all the required information to expedite your approval process?

11. Is the facility where the operation is performed set up to deal with obese patients? Those that are will have wide wheelchairs, large hospital gowns, and special tables and equipment—all designed to maximize your comfort and reduce the embarrassment you might feel being in such a vulnerable situation. This is actually one of the criteria for being designated a Center of Excellence, but you may get a sense of whether you like the place by the *tone* of the answer.

Once you feel comfortable that you've chosen the right facility or surgeon, there's the pre-op protocol. Some surgeons will ask you to lose weight before the surgery, and perhaps to consume only liquids for two to three weeks prior to the operation for a total of about one thousand calories a day. That helps to shrink the liver, which must be moved during the procedure in order to get to the stomach and place the band. If the liver is too large and plump, reaching the stomach is harder, and sometimes impossible, and often means more time under anesthesia than should have been necessary.

Also part of the pre-op protocol, common to all bariatric practices, will be general tests such as those performed before any surgery, including blood tests, a urine test, and a chest X-ray or an electrocardiogram. The surgeon's office will either do these screenings or want a copy of them from your own physician. You may also need to have your gastrointestinal tract examined with X-rays or a fluoroscope (a video that acts like a series of X-rays).

And if you have sleep apnea and use a continuous positive airway pressure (C-PAP) machine, you'll be advised to bring it to the hospital on the day of the operation so the nurses can apply it while you are sleeping after the surgery. Likewise, anyone with diabetes will have to get blood sugar in good control before undergoing this elective surgery.

Here is our own protocol for accepting patients for banding at the New York University Program for Surgical Weight Loss. Most others tend to be quite similar, with, for the most part, only slight variations here and there.

1. *Determine whether your weight makes surgery an option for you.* You have to be at least one hundred pounds overweight *or* have a BMI over forty *or* a BMI over thirty-five with health problems related to obesity. You also have to have tried medically supervised dieting but been unsuccessful at keeping off any lost weight.

You'll find a BMI chart on pages 102 and 103. Generally speaking, a BMI under 25 is considered healthy weight; a BMI from 25 to 29 is overweight; a BMI of 30 to 34 is obese; 35 to 40, severely obese; and 40 or higher, morbidly obese. At five feet nine inches and 325 pounds, Khaliah was morbidly obese.

2. *Attend a free information session.* At many hospitals, either a surgeon, nurse, or dietitian will present the surgical options for obesity—usually a gastric band or gastric bypass, explaining what they're about and detailing what living with a band is like. We also recommend attending a monthly support group, if one is available. Often run by a social worker, it's free and will help prospective candidates gear up for the operation.

3. *Determine how you will pay for the surgery.* If you are planning to pay out of pocket, the financial end is obviously uncomplicated.

If you are planning to have your surgery paid for by insurance, the first thing to do is call your insurance carrier and make sure your plan provides coverage for weight-loss surgery and that you have covered benefits for treatment of morbid obesity.

Whether private insurers pay for obesity surgery varies widely from state in state. In New York, for instance, 90 percent of insurance companies will pay for bariatric surgery, including band surgery. In Florida, none will pay. Private insurance coverage *is* expected to become more consistent, in no small part because Medicare announced last year that it would pay for bariatric surgery, including gastric banding, as long as the operation is performed at a fully qualified hospital. But for now, you need to do a little insurance homework before committing.

Assuming your insurance company will pick up the tab, the person you speak to there may ask for the name of the surgery and the diagnosis code, known in the insurance industry as the CPT/ICD-9 code. The name of the surgery is laparoscopic gastric banding (#43770), and the diagnosis code for morbid obesity is 278.01.

Be sure to get the name of the person you speak with—first name, last name, and direct phone number. This is important because your call to the insurance company may be for informational purposes only. The surgery authorization process is often actually initiated at the surgeon's office, and staff there will need to know your initial contact.

Note that in some cases, the billing coordinator at the hospital cannot initiate your surgery authorization process until you have a surgery date, which comes late in the process of being accepted for the operation, perhaps after you've had a consultation with your surgeon. While the sequence of not getting insurance authorization until you have a surgery date may seem out of order, if you initiate your surgery authorization process with-

BODY MASS INDEX TABLE

To use the table, find the appropriate height in the left-hand column labeled Height. *Move across to a given weight (in pounds). The number at the top of the column is the BMI at that height and weight. Pounds have been rounded off.*

	Healthy Weight					Overweight				Obese							Severely Obese	
BMI	19	20	21	22	23	24	25	26	27	28	29	30	31	32	33	34	35	36
Height (inches)	Body Weight (pounds)																	
58	91	96	100	105	110	115	119	124	129	134	138	143	148	153	158	162	167	172
59	94	99	104	109	114	119	124	128	133	138	143	148	153	158	163	168	173	178
60	97	102	107	112	118	123	128	133	138	143	148	153	158	163	168	174	179	184
61	100	106	111	116	122	127	132	137	143	148	153	158	164	169	174	180	185	190
62	104	109	115	120	126	131	136	142	147	153	158	164	169	175	180	186	191	196
63	107	113	118	124	130	135	141	146	152	158	163	169	175	180	186	191	197	203
64	110	116	122	128	134	140	145	151	157	163	169	174	180	186	192	197	204	209
65	114	120	126	132	138	144	150	156	162	168	174	180	186	192	198	204	210	216
66	118	124	130	136	142	148	155	161	167	173	179	186	192	198	204	210	216	223
67	121	127	134	140	146	153	159	166	172	178	185	191	198	204	211	217	223	230
68	125	131	138	144	151	158	164	171	177	184	190	197	203	210	216	223	230	236
69	128	135	142	149	155	162	169	176	182	189	196	203	209	216	223	230	236	243
70	132	139	146	153	160	167	174	181	188	195	202	209	216	222	229	236	243	250
71	136	143	150	157	165	172	179	186	193	200	208	215	222	229	236	243	250	257
72	140	147	154	162	169	177	184	191	199	206	213	221	228	235	242	250	258	265
73	144	151	159	166	174	182	189	197	204	212	219	227	235	242	250	257	265	272
74	148	155	163	171	179	186	194	202	210	218	225	233	241	249	256	264	272	280
75	152	160	168	176	184	192	200	208	216	224	232	240	248	256	264	272	279	287
76	156	164	172	180	189	197	205	213	221	230	238	246	254	263	271	279	287	295

out seeing your surgeon first and being cleared for a sur gery date, your insurance company may close your authorization case. Once you do have a scheduled surgery date, obtaining approval from your insurance carrier can take anywhere from two weeks to two months, sometimes longer. That's okay. You need

	Severely Obese									Morbidly Obese								
BMI	37	38	39	40	41	42	43	44	45	46	47	48	49	50	51	52	53	54
Height (inches)	Body Weight (pounds)																	
58	177	181	186	191	196	201	205	210	215	220	224	229	234	239	244	248	253	258
59	183	188	193	198	203	208	212	217	222	227	232	237	242	247	252	257	262	267
60	189	194	199	204	209	215	220	225	230	235	240	245	250	255	261	266	271	276
61	195	201	206	211	217	222	227	232	238	243	248	254	259	264	269	275	280	285
62	202	207	213	218	224	229	235	240	246	251	256	262	267	273	278	284	289	295
63	208	214	220	225	231	237	242	248	254	259	265	270	278	282	287	293	299	304
64	215	221	227	232	238	244	250	256	262	267	273	279	285	291	296	302	308	314
65	222	228	234	240	246	252	258	264	270	276	282	288	294	300	306	312	318	324
66	229	235	241	247	253	260	266	272	278	284	291	297	303	309	315	322	328	334
67	236	242	249	255	261	268	274	280	287	293	299	306	312	319	325	331	338	344
68	243	249	256	262	269	276	282	289	295	302	308	315	322	328	335	341	348	354
69	250	257	263	270	277	284	291	297	304	311	318	324	331	338	345	351	358	365
70	257	264	271	278	285	292	299	306	313	320	327	334	341	348	355	362	369	376
71	265	272	279	286	293	301	308	315	322	329	338	343	351	358	365	372	379	386
72	272	279	287	294	302	309	316	324	331	338	346	353	361	368	375	383	390	397
73	280	288	295	302	310	318	325	333	340	348	355	363	371	378	386	393	401	408
74	287	295	303	311	319	326	334	342	350	358	365	373	381	389	396	404	412	420
75	295	303	311	319	327	335	343	351	359	367	375	383	391	399	407	415	423	431
76	304	312	320	328	336	344	353	361	369	377	385	394	402	410	418	426	435	443

time to prepare, both emotionally and physically, and your operation can always be scheduled for a later date, if need be.

In the event that your insurance carrier denies coverage, even after an appeal, you can check into the possibility of a payment plan with the hospital's billing coordinator. Or perhaps you could get help from one of the following:

* Vocational Rehabilitation Services (www.jan.wvu.edu/ SBSES/VOCREHAB.HTM). You can find the local office in the government pages of the phone book. They may offer financial assistance to help gain or maintain employment, which may include assistance for surgery.

* Care Credit (www.carecredit.com), or call 800-859-9975.

* Patient Financial Services (www.p-f-s.com), or call 888-737-3679.

Capital One's Cosmetic Fee Plan (888-440-2375; www .cosmeticfeeplan.com), may also be able to help. And the company that makes the band currently used in the United States, Allergan, helps people pay for the surgery in monthly installments by making arrangements with various banks (877-527-2263, X4).

4. *Organize your medical records.* Whether you pay for your surgery out of pocket or through your health insurance plan, you must generally get the following to your surgeon's office: your patient information profile (we provide the form); a letter from your primary care physician, on letterhead, stating that he or she recommends you for weight-loss surgery; a complete referral from your physician that

includes a standard blood test (with blood cell counts and a comprehensive metabolic panel, liver panel, and a test for thyroid hormone); a recent photograph; documentation of at least six months of weight-loss attempt under a physician's supervision (which Khaliah, too, had to supply); and a medical history and record of a physical exam from your primary care physician, including any of your co-morbidities (such as high blood pressure or diabetes).

5. *Meet with the psychologist.* Because surgical weight loss is such a serious decision, it is important to make sure you are ready for the changes in your lifestyle that it will bring—eating much less, eating much more slowly, and not being able to turn to food when you are anxious or frustrated because it will no longer fit down your stomach. That is why clearance from a psychologist is required. Virtually all bariatric surgery practices require some type of psychiatric screening.

6. *Schedule a nutritional assessment and evaluation.* Once you have met with the psychologist, you must call the surgeon's office to schedule an appointment with the dietitian on staff and also to see one of the nurses. You must bring to the appointment everything you've pulled together in organizing your medical records.

During the visit, the dietitian will conduct a nutritional assessment and review the presurgery eating plan with you. Specifically, for two weeks prior to the surgery, you will be on a liquid diet that allows one thousand calories a day and at least fifty grams of protein. The bulk of those calories will come from meal replacement shakes. You will also be permitted to eat low-calorie vegetables such as broccoli and spinach (not starchy ones like potatoes) in small portions at lunch and dinner.

After you meet with the dietitian, the nurse will meet with you for a complete history and physical. It's somewhat redundant, since your primary care physician has already done that, but many obesity surgeons, including us, want to get certain questions answered for ourselves and also go over any questions you may have regarding the surgery. At that point the hospital staff may discuss with you the opportunity to access EMMI (www.emmi.com), an acronym for Expectation Management and Medical Information. That's a Web-based presurgical education tool that will help answer questions and familiarize you better with the whole process.

> **7.** *Schedule a surgical consultation.* Once you have been cleared by the psychologist, you may call to make an appointment for a consultation with your surgeon. (At NYU, you must be accompanied by a family member or other partner on the day of your consultation.) Only your surgeon can clear you for the operation. You will not be given a surgery date until one of us has met with you and given the go-ahead.

If this all seems like a lot of rigmarole, it is. It's important that you go through the paces not only because the health screening is crucial to determine your body's readiness for surgery but also to ensure both to yourself and to us that you are ready to make the lifestyle commitment necessary to living thin. Keep in mind that after a lifetime of using food in so many ways other than as a source of energy, eating simply for physical sustenance can be a major adjustment.

Having said that, we in no way mean to discourage people

from eligibility for gastric banding. In fact, if you are not accepted for surgery on the first go-round, we or our staff will help you prepare for a more successful follow-up evaluation. Our aim is not to exclude and sift patients out but to work with them to include them as viable candidates. No one is automatically stamped with a permanent *No.*

Once you are cleared for surgery, the Department of Surgery at the NYU Medical Center offers, free, a book and audiocassette entitled *Prepare for Surgery, Heal Faster.* Written by Peggy Huddleston and incorporating techniques that are now used at hospitals across the United States, they teach the skill of deep relaxation in order to reduce anxiety and feel calm. Feeling peaceful both soothes the nervous system and strengthens the immune system. It also balances the endocrine (hormone) and cardiovascular systems, enhancing overall healing after an operation. Finally, it can help reduce postsurgical pain and pain medication needs, decrease the length of a hospital stay, and reduce high blood pressure.

Along with the book and tape, you are welcome to participate in a one-hour workshop and telephone support. Ideally, you will start the *Heal* program one to two weeks before your operation.

Frequently Asked Questions

Khaliah had only a few questions before her surgery, but there are a number of others that prospective patients often ask.

a) How soon will I start to lose weight?

You will start losing weight immediately. With a gastric band, the loss is gradual and constant, approximately one to two pounds a week.

b) Is it possible for me to get too thin?

It is highly unusual for someone to become too thin after banding surgery because we can control how much weight you lose either by tightening or loosening the band.

c) What are the risks of the surgery?

Potential banding candidates have to be aware that electing to have an operation is a major decision and is not without some risks, which, while extremely rare, can occur. These include accidental perforation of the stomach, liver, or spleen; blood clots in the legs (deep vein thrombosis) that can sometimes migrate to the lungs or heart (pulmonary embolus); infections; partially (and temporarily) collapsed lungs; bleeding; band slippage; band erosion; and related complications that, once in two thousand times, prove fatal.

d) What if I want to get pregnant?

Simply have some or all of the fluid removed from the band (via a simple outpatient procedure that takes a few minutes in the office) to allow it to slacken so you can take in enough nutrients during your pregnancy. After delivery (or after breast-feeding), the band can be retightened with an injection of more fluid.

e) What will happen to the excess skin after I lose weight?

Some people find such skin a nuisance or cosmetically unappealing. Others do not. If you decide on plastic surgery to remove excess skin folds, be aware that it is not covered by insurance. However, many plastic surgeons are flexible and may be able to work out a payment schedule with you.

f) When will I be able to return to work or exercise?

Most people can go back to work within a week, sometimes less. You should begin to perform normal activities as soon as you feel ready. For some people, this is as early as one week postsurgery. However, no exercise or heavy exertion/lifting for at least four weeks.

g) Can I regain weight?

As we told Khaliah, you can. While the band both removes hunger and provides constant restriction, you can still eat around it. Soft, highly caloric sweets like chocolate and ice cream can slip through the tiny opening left by the band, as can high-calorie beverages such as soda pop and shakes. Keep sipping on those, even though you won't be hungry for them, and you will gain weight. Don't worry, though. Most people are so elated by their lack of hunger and the ease with which they can turn down food that the last thing they would do is go out of their way to sabotage their own efforts.

6

CHANGING MY SAIL

The alarm clock rang at 3:15 A.M., and my mother and I were on the road by four. It was pitch-black out, with no other cars around, and the surreal eeriness heightened what I can only describe as an unpleasant and unnerving combination of tension and fatigue. But my mood lightened when we crossed Dutton Mill Road, a street not too far from my house.

Fifteen years earlier, the ex-wife of my mother's older brother Kelly called one day to say she had made millions of dollars and bought a home on that road and that we should come to see it. In her head, she had been cashing in on one of her crazy get-rich-quick schemes, even though in reality no such dream was materializing.

When my mother and I arrived, I started laughing so hard that the realtor thought I was crazy. It was a large, amazing house worth millions—a compound, really—and my onetime aunt was trying to explain that her ship had come in and that she would soon be taking possession of it. The place even had a name, Château Something-or-Other, but my mother and I dubbed it Château Le Donkey Fly, meaning that our erstwhile relative would be able to afford such a dwelling when donkeys flew.

From then on, Dutton Mill Road always reminded us of our made-up Le Donkey Fly expression, but that morning, the silly idiom took on a new meaning. Crossing that road meant the donkey really had flown; I was going to be doing the impossible, getting my weight down once and for all.

For the remainder of the drive, I felt at ease. My mother fell asleep, and I listened to my meditation tape, then put on the Chaka Khan CD with my song. Around the Newark Airport exit on the New Jersey Turnpike, the sun started to rise, and I felt happy. It was a transition, a passage. A calm came over me, even though I was experiencing a strong rush of excitement.

I thought a lot about a saying I had heard once: "You can't change the wind, but you can change your sail." I felt that's what was going on. I wasn't able to change the course of nature—all the things in my life and my makeup that had contributed to my obesity—but I was now going to change the sail. That is, I was going to alter my *response* to the wind that had blown my way.

I was going over in my head every diet book I ever read, every walk I ever took to Weight Watchers, every grapefruit and boiled egg I'd ever stuffed down. It had all led to this moment, I felt. I appeared to have found the way.

Then we glided into Manhattan. There was not an ounce of traffic, a New York miracle in itself, but as the car headed east toward First Avenue, I saw the big, cold gray hospital building, and I was scared all over again. The down-on-the-ground reality of the operation hit me once more.

I woke my mother and called Peggy Tagliarino, the public relations agent for Drs. Fielding and Ren. "Get yourself together because the camera crews are ready and waiting," she said.

She was right, of course. I had known in advance that the *Today* show was going to be covering the whole procedure, from pre-op to the aftermath, so I had to gear up not just for the operation but also for filming. I had promised Drs. Fielding and Ren that I would help publicize banding as an alternative to gastric bypass.

Once I parked the car, I called my mother's husband, a high school principal she had married several years earlier, a man who is very good to both her and her family. Jacob wasn't up yet, he said, which frustrated me because I was hoping to say hello to him before all the hubbub started.

Then I began to feel nervous about the solids I had eaten over the last two weeks. It had been nagging at me, and now my dietary transgressions loomed large. Would my liver be too big to perform the operation? Should I say something to Dr. Fielding?

There wasn't any time to get bogged down in remorse, though. As soon as I went up the elevator, I was met by a publicist from NYU Medical Center, the *Today* camera crew, and Peggy. The show was going on, it *must* go on—there was no turning back—and it was being filmed for posterity.

I was led back through a hallway to fill out all the pre-op paperwork, then taken upstairs to the operating-room floor. My heart felt as though it was beating right through my chest to the outside, like in a cartoon.

Fortunately, the cameras stopped rolling for a while at that point, and warmth followed. Some wonderful nurses came over, holding my hand and speaking to me in soothing tones while giving me my hospital gown. Gaspar Rosario, my favorite nurse of all, gave me a huge, everything's-going-to-be-okay hug.

Afterward, they weighed me. One final mortifying clanking of the metal weights over all those numbers on the vertical hospital scale. Heavy as ever, I thought to myself that I was never going to be able to lose all this weight. It seemed too easy.

It was at that point that the *Today* show wanted to know if they could film me in my gown. That *was* easy. The answer was no.

I was soon walked over to another area, and then, through a set of double doors came the surgeons, looking like superheroes. Dr. Fielding was handsome and confident, as usual. Dr. Ren had on skintight white pants with an eyelet design cut into them, plus a tight little white blazer. I remember thinking, okay, they can cut into me, fly me over the danger to safety.

As soon as I looked at Dr. Fielding, he came over to me, and my fears truly did go out the window. I really had put all my trust in him. After that, the staff couldn't get me into the OR fast enough; I was actually feeling impatient and wanted to get going.

Dr. Fielding left for a short time, and I used the opportunity to make a few phone calls to my son. I was speaking to him on and off until about five minutes before I went into the operating room. He was glad enough to hear from me but kept wanting to go back to watching *Scooby-Doo*, which was exactly as I wished it. I wanted him distracted rather than missing me, which freed me up.

I don't know how much sense I was making toward the end, anyway. One of the nurses gave me a short-acting Valium to relax me, and I started getting silly. "Don't show my arms," I said to the film crew. "Don't tuck all my hair up into my cap; I need some of it sticking out. I need a little bit of makeup on." I was playing prima donna, joking around and even dancing a little.

Then they rolled me in, and Dr. Fielding came over—he had

changed into his scrubs—and told me I had nothing to worry about. "There's nothing in this world that I love doing more," he said. "You're in safe hands."

I knew at that moment that I needed to decide whether to tell him about the solid foods I had sneaked here and there over the last two weeks. I opted against it. It was a gamble, I knew. But I had come almost the whole distance; I couldn't bear the thought of not being able to follow through with this.

Before going under, I looked around me and was amazed at what I saw. Dr. Fielding's surgical team was a rainbow of colors. A Dr. Duane Fredericks from Guyana was assisting; Gio Dugay, a nurse practitioner from the Philippines, popped in to give me one last reassurance; and Gaspar, who is from the Dominican Republic, was also on hand. The anesthesiologist was Israeli, with a thick accent. The diversity made me cry. I was overwhelmed by a strong feeling of pride, and felt very clearly that I had chosen right by choosing Dr. Fielding. I was proud and happy.

A couple of moments later I put my life into the hands of everyone in that room. The anesthesiologist told me to count backward from ten, and as I started, I took one last look at the clock. It was a little after 7 A.M., the same time of day I had been born, and here I was once again pushing through something to the other side . . .

GASTRIC BANDING VERSUS OTHER WEIGHT-LOSS SURGERIES: THE NUTS AND BOLTS

Gastric banding is our surgery of choice for most overweight people. It's the safest and, over the long term, just as effective as more risk-laden procedures. But it is not the only kind of bariatric operation we perform. On the contrary, many of the two hundred thousand people in the United States who undergo weight-loss operations each year still opt for other types of procedures, in large part because they don't know about the band.

The most common type of weight-loss surgery performed in the United States (though not in the world) is **gastric bypass**. It's also known as a Roux-En Y. The *Roux* is for Caesar Roux, the French surgeon who first described the intestinal rearrangement the operation entails. And the *Y* is for the way your intestines look after the procedure.

With a gastric bypass, food literally bypasses most of the stomach. In fact, the surgeon performs the first part of the operation by closing off and disconnecting 95 percent of the stomach with a stapling device. What could once stretch to the size of a football is reduced to the size of an egg that can hold, at most, only a couple of tablespoons of food.

Following the stomach reduction, the surgeon cuts the small intestine into two pieces. The lower piece, two to three feet down from the upper piece, is then connected to the newly created, tiny stomach pouch, leaving the upper part of the intestine out of the picture. That's significant because much of our nutrient absorption takes place in the small intestine. If several feet of it are bypassed, that means fewer nutrients are absorbed, particularly protein, calcium, and iron.

The upshot: not only does less food fit into the newly created tiny stomach pouch, which makes a person feel full on much less food than before, but fewer of that food's nutrients make their way into the body's cells.

Advantages of Gastric Bypass: People who have undergone gastric bypass lose, on average, 60 to 80 percent of their

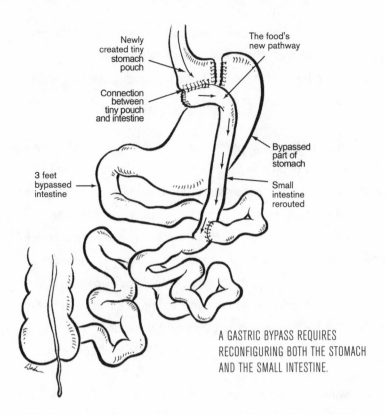

Newly created tiny stomach pouch

The food's new pathway

Connection between tiny pouch and intestine

Bypassed part of stomach

3 feet bypassed intestine

Small intestine rerouted

A GASTRIC BYPASS REQUIRES RECONFIGURING BOTH THE STOMACH AND THE SMALL INTESTINE.

excess body weight within two years. And their health conditions are either greatly improved or even resolved. Diabetes, high blood pressure, sleep apnea, high cholesterol—they all become much less severe or go away entirely.

Disadvantages of Gastric Bypass: The surgery is by no means risk-free. As many as four in one hundred patients suffer, and sometimes die, from such complications as leakage of intestinal fluid into the abdominal cavity within weeks of the operation. Imagine stapling together two pieces of paper, or sewing two pieces of cloth. Sometimes a staple pops off or a stitch tears. Similarly, after gastric bypass surgery, the staples (which are small, permanent, and made of titanium) may pop, or stitches may tear, causing a small hole in the stomach or intestine.

Digestive juices or bile could seep out through one of the holes and cause a serious infection known as peritonitis.

Other life-threatening possibilities: blood clots that start in the legs and can travel to the lungs; heart attack; or respiratory failure.

Another problem for gastric bypass patients—all of them—is malabsorption of nutrients. Since part of the small intestine is bypassed, it is difficult, if not impossible, to get enough protein, calcium, and certain vitamins. For that reason, people who have undergone gastric bypass must take vitamin and mineral supplements every single day for the rest of their lives. These include a multivitamin, calcium, vitamin B_{12}, and iron. They also need to work closely with a dietitian to make sure that the small amount of food they are taking in contains enough protein. Blood tests may be performed every three months for the first year to check nutritional status.

Yet another issue for many people who have had gastric bypass: transient hair loss. Eighty to 90 percent of bypass patients lose significant amounts of their hair at first, when their bodies are not yet used to the rapid weight loss. Regrowth does not typically occur until after about six months.

Gallstones are common in gastric bypass patients, too, as is lactose intolerance. Lactase, the enzyme that helps break down milk products, doesn't enter the digestive system at the same place anymore, so milk-based items are more prone to cause gas, belching, diarrhea, and other GI upset.

Then there's the dumping syndrome, which can occur after eating just one bite of something sugary (and, in some cases, greasy). High-sugar foods move quickly from the stomach to the small intestine, and that rapid transit time can lead to a variety of unpleasant symptoms the moment the sugar (or fat) contacts the intestine. These include sweating, nausea, faintness, diarrhea, cramps, and rapid pulse.

The dumping syndrome can be considered a disadvantage or an advantage, depending on how you look at it. It's a disadvantage from the point of view of feeling lousy, but an advantage in that it conditions people against eating sweets. That said, not all gastric bypass patients experience dumping, and many who do experience it do so only for the first year or two, so you should not have that surgery counting on the dumping syndrome to keep you from eating pastries, candy, ice cream, and the like.

Also important to think about when considering gastric bypass is the fact that, for all practical purposes, the operation is irreversible. There is a greatly increased chance of complications from excess scar tissue that could form as a result of a second operation in the same area.

Then, too, evidence is coming to light that in rare cases, people who undergo gastric bypass, while resolving their diabetes, end up with blood sugar that sporadically falls too *low,* a condition known as hypoglycemia. In some instances, blood sugar goes low enough to cause blackouts, increasing the risk for car accidents and such (it has already happened).

It appears that after gastric bypass, the pancreas can essentially go into overdrive, producing too much of the hormone insulin, which allows sugar to be removed from the bloodstream. Too much insulin secreted, too little sugar in the blood.

Finally, some weight regain with gastric bypass generally occurs. The stomach softens up after a while, allowing more food in with less discomfort. There is no adjustment that can be made to retighten it.

A second type of weight-loss surgery available in the United States is the **biliopancreatic diversion**. Like gastric bypass, it bypasses part of the small intestine and reconnects it in a Y configuration. But it leaves more of the stomach intact by removing two-thirds of it rather than bypassing 95 percent, as in gastric bypass, so that what is left is the size of a banana. Yet some fifteen feet of intestine are bypassed, as opposed to just two to three feet with gastric bypass. Thus, this operation is less about being able to hold a small amount of food in your stomach and much more about poor absorption of nutrients, most importantly, calories. (The reason it's called biliopancreatic diversion is that bile from

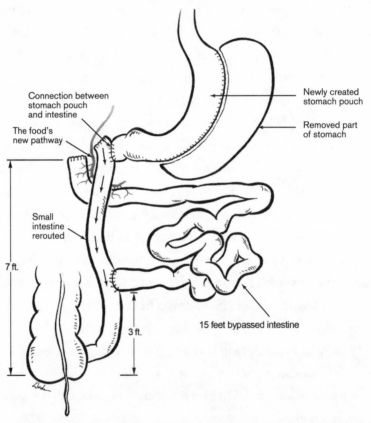

A BILIOPANCREATIC DIVERSION BYPASSES FIFTEEN FEET OF THE INTESTINE. THE INTESTINE IS WHERE SO MANY OF OUR NUTRIENTS ARE ABSORBED. (THE TYPE OF BILIOPANCREATIC DIVERSION PICTURED HERE IS KNOWN AS A DUODENAL SWITCH.)

the liver and digestive enzymes from the pancreas are diverted to the lower end of the small intestine rather than hitting food at the upper end.)

Advantages of Biliopancreatic Diversion: The pounds lost after the operation average 70 to 90 percent of excess body weight over the first two years, with virtually no regain. There is generally no dumping syndrome, either. The larger stomach size means food empties from the stomach into the small intestine more slowly, doing away with the rapid transit time that causes all the unpleasant symptoms.

Disadvantages of Biliopancreatic Diversion: Once this operation is performed, only 25 percent of all fat eaten is absorbed; 75 percent is "pooped out." Nonabsorbed fat means most patients experience frequent, foul-smelling, pasty bowel movements, especially after eating fatty food. Associated side effects include flatulence and bloating. These effects may improve after the first six months.

Also, since more of the food eaten goes unabsorbed, there is a tenfold greater chance for nutritional deficiencies than with gastric bypass. In addition to the supplements mentioned in the discussion about gastric bypass, patients must take, every single day for the rest of their lives, vitamins A, D, E, and K. (These are fat-soluble, meaning they are absorbed efficiently only in the presence of sufficient dietary fat. Without enough fat, supplemental doses are required.)

Finally, because the stomach pouch ends up larger than with gastric bypass, there is concern among some people that biliopancreatic diversion patients will end up with more acid and therefore are more apt to experience heartburn. There is also a small chance that they will develop ulcers in the small intestine and therefore need to take antiulcer medication after surgery.

Note that biliopancreatic diversion is no surgical walk in the park. While a gastric bypass operation takes about two to three hours and requires a two- to three-day hospital stay, *this* operation takes up to five hours and requires up to five days in the hospital. And certain variations on the procedure carry an even greater risk of life-threatening intestinal leakage than gastric bypass does.

We don't perform biliopancreatic diversions anymore because there are just too many downsides, particularly the lifelong nutritional deficiencies. Of the surgeons in the United States who do perform the surgery, only a handful perform it laparoscopically. Laparoscopic surgery means the surgeon gets to the internal organs simply by making about a half-dozen tiny cuts (all less

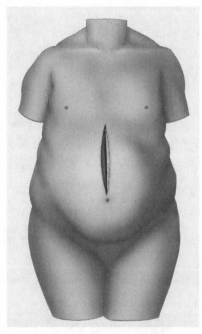

OPEN SURGERY INCISION. WITH OPEN SURGERY, A SIX-INCH-LONG CUT IS REQUIRED.
Courtesy Allergan Medical.

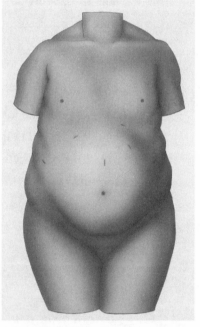

PERFORMED LAPAROSCOPICALLY, GASTRIC BANDING REQUIRES ONLY FIVE OR SIX TINY INCISIONS, EACH LESS THAN A HALF INCH LONG.
Courtesy Allergan Medical.

than a half inch long) in the abdomen and then watching the patient's insides on television monitors as he or she moves various surgical instruments where they need to be. (A tiny camera is inserted through one of the cuts, which allows the images to be projected onto a screen.) But most surgeons who perform this operation in North America use conventional surgery—a six-inch or larger incision required for looking at the stomach and intestine directly. The larger incision means more postoperative pain, longer healing time, and a higher risk of infection, blood clots, pneumonia, and hernias.

Almost all **gastric banding surgeries,** by contrast, are performed via laparoscopy (as are more and more gastric bypass operations), greatly improving the safety of the procedure, and greatly ratcheting down the pain and recovery time. You might assume that on some level, it's better to conduct an operation looking directly at the organs you're operating on, even if that creates a bigger wound. But that's not the case. Consider that the camera systems used in laparoscopic surgery are so sophisticated that it's as if the surgeon's eye is right up against the tissue, rather than looking at it from above. Moreover, many operating rooms, like ours, are now like video-game parlors, with up to five screens in order to allow everyone in the OR, not just the surgeon, to see what is going on, which makes it easier to assist.

The nitty-gritty of banding surgery is as follows. Through one of the tiny laparoscopic cuts in your abdomen, a hollow tube is inserted that allows carbon dioxide to be pumped inside and thereby create a large space; your belly becomes about the same size as it would be in the third trimester of pregnancy. That gives the surgeon enough room to do all the necessary work (all the gas is released at the end of the operation, and you instantly resume your preoperative shape).

The surgeon then inserts hollow tubes called trocars into your abdomen in various locations. The trocars allow long surgical instruments to reach your gastrointestinal tract so the surgeon can manipulate your stomach and the organs around it without actually touching them. The full vision offered by the television screens is what allows the work to be so precise. Think of it as the surgeon playing the piano without looking down at his or her hands while at the same time performing as a slick video-game master. (Laparoscopy will come easily to those in the Play-Station generation who grow up to be surgeons someday.)

Beside the advantage that gastric banding has of virtually always being performed laparoscopically (unless, for instance, a complication like a too-large liver requires conversion to conventional surgery—with a large incision—while the patient is on the table), it does not result in nutrient malabsorption, as do gastric bypass and biliopancreatic diversion. It is strictly about restricting the amount of food you can eat.

A silicone band (hard silicone, not the liquid silicone used in breast implants) is wrapped around the upper part of the stomach, then locked much the way a belt is locked. That creates a small stomach pouch with an opening to the rest of the stomach that is about a half inch wide—the size of your thumbnail. Food passes through the opening to the bottom of the stomach very slowly, resulting in feeling full longer.

The width of the narrowing can be adjusted to decrease hunger, or increase it, say, for pregnancy. That's because the inner surface of the band contains a balloon that can be inflated or deflated with a completely nontoxic watery solution (think of sterile salt water, like what people rinse their contact lenses with). The water modifies the size of the opening. The more water in the band, the more narrow the opening.

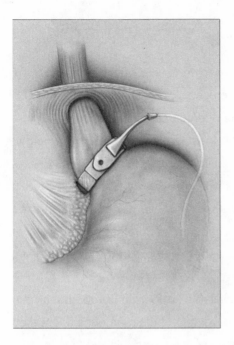

THE GASTRIC BAND IN PLACE NEAR THE TOP OF THE STOMACH. Courtesy Allergan Medical.

How, exactly, does the amount of water in the band get adjusted? The band is connected to a strawlike tube, about a foot long, that is placed in the abdomen during the surgery. The tube, in turn, is connected to a reservoir that the surgeon also places in the abdomen during the operation. (The reservoir cannot be seen, only felt, when you push on your abdomen.) At any point in time after the operation, the surgeon can control the amount of water in the band by passing a water-filled needle into the skin, and from there into the reservoir, where the water is then injected and heads from the reservoir into the tube and up into the silicone-surrounded balloon. The injection either inserts more water (tightening the opening between the upper and lower stomach) or withdraws water (loosening of the band, say, for pregnancy). You never have to worry that the needle will go in too deep. The reservoir has a rubber top that makes the needle easy to inject, but a metal floor that the needle could never pass through.

While gastric banding was approved in the United States in 2001 and is still only rarely used here, accounting for just one in five U.S weight-loss surgeries, it has been standard procedure in Europe since 1994. In fact, it is the most commonly performed weight-loss operation outside the United States. In Italy, the surgery is free, paid for by the national health insurance plan. It's covered in France, too. And requirements for how overweight you have to be to qualify are becoming less stringent in Europe because the procedure is deemed so safe, especially next to the risks of being very overweight.

The surgery is readily available not only in Europe but also in Australia, the Middle East, Mexico, and Latin America. More than two hundred thousand severely obese people worldwide have had a band inserted.

Advantages of Gastric Banding Surgery, also known as Laparoscopic Adjustable Gastric Banding: Weight loss during the first three years ranges from 50 to 65 percent of excess body weight, reducing or completely resolving complications from such conditions as diabetes, heart disease, and osteoarthritis, just like

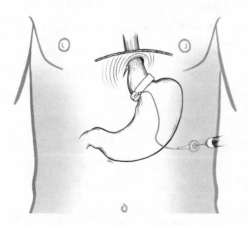

FLUID IS INJECTED TO (OR WITHDRAWN FROM) THE BAND FOR TIGHTENING (OR LOOSENING) WITH A NEEDLE IN A SIMPLE OFFICE VISIT.

the other surgeries. Granted, the number of pounds shed in the first three years is somewhat less dramatic than with gastric bypass or biliopancreatic diversion, but there's a big difference. Pretty much *all* the weight loss with those other operations occurs within the first two years, generally within even the first eighteen months. The surgery in those cases is the beginning and the end of the solution. Weight loss with a gastric band, on the other hand, can go on for much longer because you can always have the band retightened. Three to five years out, weight-loss results with a band are just as impressive as with other types of weight-loss surgery.

Research out of Australia that looked at results on almost twenty-four thousand weight-loss surgery patients proved it. Pound for pound, gastric bypass beat the band for the first three years, but a few years after that, the banded patients caught up.

In the United States, a gastric band achieves the same amount of weight loss as gastric bypass at three years. But either way, the slower weight loss granted by the band is easier on the body, and also gives the patient more time to adjust to a new way of eating that will be healthful throughout his or her life.

Gastric banding is also the least invasive of all bariatric surgeries available. There's no cutting or reconnecting of the stomach or small intestine. Thus, *there is also virtually no risk with a band of life-threatening intestinal leakage, dumping, or other food intolerance.* That's a large part of the reason the death rate from bandng surgery is one in two thousand as opposed to one in two hundred from the other types of surgery.

And the surgery is 100 percent reversible. If, for whatever reason, you no longer want the band, you can have it removed.

Disadvantages of Gastric Banding: The success of the band is 70 percent dependent on your commitment to follow up with your surgeon every six to eight weeks for at least the first year. Close monitoring of your rate of weight loss, eating habits, and various symptoms will determine whether you need a band adjustment. Of course, the frequent contact with your surgeon may also be viewed as an advantage. More follow-up care with your doctor is going to improve your chances of losing weight as quickly as possible and learning to eat more healthfully in the bargain.

Worth bearing in mind is that because the band is an implantable device, it does carry the risk of slippage (causing complete blockage between the upper and lower parts of the stomach) or erosion into the stomach (causing weight loss to stop). In either case, a second laparoscopic surgery would be required to reposition the band (if it has slipped) or remove it (if it has eroded). Such complications are exceedingly rare, but they do happen.

Finally, as we stated in chapter five, the band will not result in weight loss if you eat around it (or more precisely, through it) by taking in too much of soft, caloric foods like chocolate or drinking too many high-calorie beverages like shakes and soda pop. These can go through the tiny opening in the band all too easily, sabotaging your efforts and all you put yourself through to have the band implanted. In other words, with a gastric band, you have to *participate* in your own weight loss. It's much, much easier than without the band, but weight loss won't just happen. The band is a tool that will let you *make* it happen.

Fortunately, people are generally so amazed by their smaller appetites, and their slimming bodies, that they want to do everything they can to work with all the gastric band has to offer. Since Dr. Fielding had his band implanted, he eats about one-sixth the volume of food he used to. Ever since he was a child, he had second helpings at meals, ending up eating five slices of meat, three potatoes, some pumpkin, a roast onion, and beans

WEIGHT-LOSS SURGERIES AT A GLANCE

	Gastric Bypass	Biliopancreatic Diversion	Gastric Banding
Length of surgery	2–3 hours	3–5 hours	1 hour
Length of hospital stay	2–3 days	4–5 days	1 day
Time off work	3 weeks	3–4 weeks	1 week or less
Reversible?	No	No	Yes
Mortality Rate	1 in 200	1 in 100	1 in 2,000
Complications:			
Intestinal leaks	(2–3%)	(3–4%)	Band slippage (3–5%)
Bleeding	(2%)	(3%)	Port or tubing problems (2%)
Intestinal blockage	(2%)	(3%)	Erosion (0.1%)
Nutrient deficiencies	(5–10%)	(60–70%)	—

and gravy. *Now* he feels full after *one* piece of fish, *one* potato, and some beans—and is too happy about his thinness to ruin it with soft solids or caloric liquids.

Indeed, there are fewer happier people on earth than formerly fat people. Maybe that's why some patients who have had the surgery even legally change their birthdays to the day of their operation. It's kind of like being born again, as Khaliah intimated.

7

A NEW DAY DAWNS

How was my liver?"

Dr. Fielding had just walked into my hospital room. I woke up shortly before that and had been looking out the window. It was very bright out, one of those rare August mornings with not a cloud in the sky but with no shimmer of humidity, either.

He had one of those smiles that a proud new father has on his face, so I assumed I'd made it through. But when I asked him my question, his expression sobered some. "Your liver was fine," he told me, but he let me know with his inflection that he understood I was confessing my lack of adherence to the liquid fast in the weeks leading up to the surgery.

"You took a chance," he said. Not adhering to the fast, he continued, could have made the operation longer, and they might have had to keep me under anesthesia a bit longer than should have been necessary because manipulating a too-big liver to get to the stomach can take a little doing.

Then he let it go. There was no finger wagging. Instead, he spoke to me encouragingly and gave me some instructions to rest and not be overambitious in my recovery. He also reminded me not to try eating any solids because I could vomit and dislodge the band, but he reassured me that I wouldn't be feeling hungry because even though the first band tightening was six weeks away, my stomach was swollen and tender, and that would kill hunger.

He was right. I hadn't eaten since six o'clock the night before, but I wasn't the least bit hungry.

Dr. Fielding left shortly thereafter, and I looked back out the window. The sunshine was dancing on the East River; it was dancing on my heart. I did it! I was both excited and curious.

Then I moved a little and felt tenderness and told myself to take it easy. At that point, my mother came into the room and kept me company while I did my hair and makeup. The *Today* show crew had long gone, but I didn't want to feel like a hospital patient.

I called Jacob—"Mom, when are you coming home?"—after which a nurse made me walk the hallway. They try to get you moving, if slowly, as soon as possible.

At about two in the afternoon, Mike Tyson's sister, Jacqueline Rowe, appeared at my door with flowers. We had met at a plus-size fashion show at Bloomingdale's a few weeks earlier, and she wanted me to know that she was thinking of me. It was one of the loveliest gestures anyone ever went out of her way to make for me.

Then there was more walking the halls with my IV drip and my mother. I was doing a lot of thinking and feeling a lot of excitement. Here I was with this new instrument in me, and I didn't even know yet what that really meant. The only thing that was clear was that I didn't feel hungry.

My cousin Ivana, herself a Ford model, came that evening and took my mother to dinner, which was fine with me because I was in and out of sleep, anyway. Also, as accommodating as NYU was, I was aching to get home to Jacob and be in my own house, so I was too antsy to have company by my bedside.

When my mother and Ivana left, I turned off the TV and all the lights and looked across the river as evening fell softly over Queens, thinking, thinking, thinking . . .

The next thing I knew, it was totally dark out, my mother was sleeping in the chair next to my bed, and I fell right back into slumber.

In the morning, a nurse woke me and got me out of bed and allowed me some ice chips, which I was thrilled about because my mouth felt dry. She then took out the IV (the only pain I had at that point could be quelled easily with Tylenol), and it was time for me to go downstairs to take the "swallow"—a dye that colors the insides of your esophagus and stomach in a way that allows an X-ray machine to make sure things are positioned inside you as they should be.

I took the elevator in my hospital gown with a group of about eight other people who had also had the surgery the day before— everyone from soccer moms to Hasidic Jews. Almost all had a family member with them, so the group as a whole came to some fifteen or twenty people.

It felt very undignified—let's herd up all the fat people (and I was one of the smaller ones there!) and take them down for their swallow. Everyone around stared at the morbidly obese bunch of us, but in a perverse sort of way, that actually made it easier. "Fine," I thought to myself. "Stare good and long. It's the last chance you'll get."

After the X-ray, I went back upstairs and quickly got out of the hospital gown and into my clothes. Dr. Fielding came by again and, in his casual Aussie style, said, "All right, mate, you did a good job. Go home. You know what to do."

When my mother and I got down to the garage, the valet handed me the car keys, and my mother shot me a look. "You're not driving," she said.

"But I can," I answered.

"You're not supposed to."

"But I can." I then drove through a good portion of Manhattan but felt too tender to drive any farther and handed the car over to my mother. I guess that's what Dr. Fielding meant about not being over-ambitious in my recovery.

When I arrived home, I already had some clear liquids in the house that I was supposed to be on for the first two weeks—consommé, diet iced tea, and so on. Jacob came over and hugged me gently—someone must have prepared him—and I surveyed the kitchen. Things were different already. I couldn't just open the fridge and make a sandwich. I couldn't pour a bowl of cereal. I wasn't at all hungry, but from now on I wasn't going to be kicking off my shoes with food, the way I usually did when I came home from somewhere.

That night, everyone was over for dinner—my mother, her husband, and my siblings. I made spaghetti with homemade meatballs, French bread, and a salad. I'm not exactly sure why, because it certainly didn't fall to me to cook the day after my procedure. I think it might have been a kind of saving face, showing that I wasn't vulnerable. But I *felt* vulnerable. While I wasn't the least bit hungry, I was so used to eating when food was around that the experience of cooking and watching everyone else dig in made me feel off-kilter.

While the others had dinner, I sucked on a Popsicle, then went upstairs to bed and did a lot of meditating and thinking. As difficult as all this was, there was something comforting about having food in front of me and not being able to eat it. Not that there was a lot of time to ruminate on it. A short time later I fell asleep, didn't awake even once during the night, and arose the next morning to more beautiful flowers from well-wishers. The good rest combined with the good wishes helped restore my emotional balance.

In my front room, I have a chair with an ottoman and a large cashmere blanket, and that's where I spent the better part of my first full day home. I would snuggle up in the blanket, read a fitness magazine or some Sri Chinmoy meditation, doze, wake up and read some more, then doze again. My mother took care of things while I relaxed.

The next day, my mother's cousin Asia, a massage therapist, came over and massaged me. After that I felt ready to get on with life, not just for my own sake but for Jacob's. I wanted him to feel that things were going on like normal, which, very soon, they were.

After one more good night's rest, Jacob and my youngest sister, Lydia, and I were off to New York so I could appear on the *Today* show with Dr. Fielding. There I was, just three days out of surgery, dragging luggage and two children through the Thirtieth Street Station in Philadelphia to catch our train to Manhattan's Penn Station. Once in New York, we checked into the Essex House Hotel, and Ivana took care of the kids while I took it easy.

I awoke for the *Today* show at four the next morning and was met downstairs by a limousine sent by NBC. As soon as I arrived at the studio, I was shuttled right to the green room. Dr. Fielding was already there, and they took us both to makeup. I felt not an ounce of nervousness.

Then we turned the corner, and I looked at the set while Matt Lauer sat at a desk explaining to viewers that they were seeing me on a gurney headed for the OR. I was nine years old again, anxious and fearful, as I had been on my first *Today* visit. But the show, as always, had to go on. Ninety seconds later, the cameras were pointed toward me, Ann Curry was asking me questions, my insides were being shown on-screen (the camera crew had filmed the actual operation), and, fortunately, confidence bypassed stage fright. Dr. Fielding and I nailed the segment, and I could tell he was proud of me, which made me so glad. Even a couple of the producers came over afterward and said I did a good job.

Soon after, I went back to the hotel, packed up, and took the kids home. This was it. I really *was* starting the rest of my life.

At first that meant more days of clear liquids—low-sodium broth, a spicy Thai soup I had found, white tea, black tea, green tea, tea derived from ayurvedic Japanese mushrooms. After two weeks of that, I was thrilled to move to the mushy food stage. I literally couldn't wait to eat cottage cheese, oatmeal. I even bought a pureeing machine and started to make my own mixtures. One of them was tuna fish mixed with green peppers, onions, carrot, and a drop of olive oil. I churned it to the same consistency as baby food, but I loved it. I also drank some yogurt concoctions at first but pulled back on those because I was worried about the calories. I did allow myself some bits of avocado, though, along with soft-boiled eggs.

Even so, this was no mushy food orgy. I had to eat much more slowly than I was used to in order not to throw up, which was very important because vomiting could make the band slip. Also, the portions were very small. Maybe half an egg or three tablespoons of the tuna concoction. I just couldn't fit any more down.

It didn't feel bad, and, again, I didn't feel hungry. To the contrary, I found the whole thing interesting, like I was my own science experiment. It was my first introduction to eating to live rather than living to eat. Taking twenty minutes to have these small meals was giving me such gratification. It was as if I could feel my body beginning to melt away. And I hadn't even started real exercise yet.

Not that I didn't do what I was able. Even from day one I walked to the mailbox. Day two I did three laps of walking around my cul-de-sac. My mother said I was being ridiculous, that I didn't need to try to move around so early in the game, but even at my heaviest, I had always engaged in at least some physical activity, so I was trying to get back to myself. "Mom, I've got to do it," I said. I was sticking with it for my emotional stability.

Fewer than four weeks after the operation, as I was about to transition from mush to solid foods, I had my first foray back into public life. The Republican convention was getting under way in New York two months before the 2004 presidential election, and an organization called People for the American Way arranged for a reading of the Constitution by celebrities in the Great Hall at Cooper Union, on East Seventh Street. The arrangers of the reading said the Constitution is a document with which Republicans "should be more familiar."

Luminaries from all walks of life were invited to read, including great entertainment figures like Lauren Bacall, Alec Baldwin, Ossie Davis, and Ruby Dee. And then there was me. I was deeply honored to be asked to read with so many people who loomed so large in their profession. It was a great moment in a young Democrat's life. But I was scared to death. While I was very thrilled to be participating in something like this while I was starting to lose weight once and for all—it boosted my confidence—I feared my dyslexia would get the better of me and that I'd screw up beyond repair. It didn't help that as I was walking in, Kathleen Turner was walking out and said to me, "This is tough." The Constitution is an intricately worded document that doesn't roll off the tongue, and with so much at stake in Iraq and after 9/11, reading our rights out loud was an emotional experience, even for a seasoned actress.

I was put in line right behind Richard Gere, which only heightened my nervousness, but I went out there and got it right—no small feat for someone who's dyslexic. I was so proud of myself. There are few occasions in my life where I'm willing to toot my own horn, but this was one of them. It was a real turning point, and I attribute its success in no small part to my operation. I felt I was truly on my way and could now do anything I set my mind to, and this was my first chance to prove it. I measured up.

There was an integrity issue, too. I wanted to give respect to what I was reading.

When I was done and leaving the building, I saw Mandy Patinkin, and the nine-year-old in me came out again. He was sitting in a stairwell I had to descend on my way out, and while I had had a major crush on him ever since he spit a cork out of his mouth in *Evita*, I couldn't bring myself to say anything and walked right past him. It was like my moments so many years earlier with Dionne Warwick. Then I said "damn it" to myself, turned around, and told him, "I have to say this. I have adored you my entire life."

He gave me a big hug. He said he was touched that I was a fan of his. I felt great, not only because he was so nice to me, but also because I conquered my fear. As soon as I was out of the building, I picked up the phone and called my mother to tell her I was just talking to Che from *Evita*, to Avigdor from *Yentl*.

A few days later, I was confronted with something unsettling enough to actually scare me. I started feeling hungry. No longer tender from the operation but two weeks shy of my first band tightening, I would find myself strolling past the Tastykakes or cheese sticks in a convenience store and *really* wanting them. It was awful, particularly because now that I was back on solid foods, it was harder for me to make sure I wasn't overeating. I was enjoying sushi again and crunchy foods like breakfast cereal. I even was able to get down a small part of an apple several days after switching back to solids. Terrified that I was going to gain weight before I had a real chance to lose any, I sweated out the time to my next appointment at the hospital. I was sure I was blowing it.

But I wasn't! When I went in for my first tightening, I had already lost sixteen pounds.

That first adjustment was really strange. I immediately felt very different. I went to drink some water in the hallway and could tell even then that something had changed. Water itself went down more slowly, more in a way that I was conscious of. "Oh my God," I said to myself. "This is working." It was true. Immediately after that first tightening, the hunger was gone, as if by the snap of someone's fingers.

I threw up my food a couple of times after the band was adjusted. I needed to learn to eat even more slowly and take even smaller bites than I had been taking. It's not like regular throw-up, where the food mixes with stomach acid and tastes sour coming back up. The food you regurgitate doesn't even make it to your stomach. It just sits on top of the band until it's ready to come back up, more or less in the form in which you swallowed it. Still, I hate throwing up, so I made sure that didn't keep happening. I paced my chewing and swallowing even beyond what initially felt normal.

It took some particular getting used to when I was eating with others, which I had to do frequently. There were still appointments to keep, business meetings, getting together with friends.

It wasn't just eating more methodically than ever that was hard. It was that people are equally quick to criticize you for not eating enough as they are for overeating. Everyone has such a critical eye that you can't win. While there's a lot of disdain for obesity and stuffing yourself, people look at you just as funny if they perceive that you're undereating.

"That's it, Khaliah?" someone would ask if I was out having a charity lunch or talking to a reporter. "I know you must be hungry."

I decided, at least at the beginning, simply not to eat in front of others. One, I didn't want to be watched; two, people tend to eat very fast, and I needed a full twenty minutes to a half hour just to get down a very small portion; and three, I just wasn't hungry. So I'd *order* a meal but basically nurse a cup of tea. (Even now when I socialize it pretty much goes that way. I've just gotten better at pushing my food around my plate, so it *seems* like I'm eating the way everyone else does.)

Two weeks after the first adjustment, when the hunger had completely dissipated because of the band tightening, I lost another six pounds, for a total of twenty-two. I couldn't believe I was losing weight, out in the world, and not suffering.

Then it was time for me to appear on *The Jane Pauley Show.* Though thrilled to have the opportunity to see her, I was not happy about the timing. The episode was entitled "Does Thinner Mean Happier?" but I hardly had a point of reference to be discussing such a topic. A loss of twenty-two pounds on a morbidly obese woman doesn't even qualify her as anywhere near half-baked.

Still, Jane was wonderful. Not that she lobbed easy questions at me. She really probed, and that, in turn, required me to be honest. But the interview was loving, and very, very warm. And that allowed me to really be in the moment. I was able to say things to her that I had waited more than twenty years to say. She showed the clip of the two of us talking when I was nine years old, and I was able to tell her, on air, that she had been my role model ever since I was a child. People in the audience were teary-eyed. A couple of the production people said they had lumps in their throats.

When it was over and time to say good-bye, she asked me how Jacob was. That meant so much to me.

It was another turning point. I was already feeling pretty sure that I was going to be able to lose a substantial amount of weight, but after that show I decided that mine was also going to be a story about health and fitness and emotional well-being. I wanted people to be able to reflect on their lives through my own experience.

Then a few more weeks passed—it was October, not even three months after the surgery—and I was down thirty-three pounds already.

Life continued to go on. I was growing my collection at Simplicity sewing patterns and beginning to gear up for launching a collection of ready-to-wear clothing in stores. I was working extensively with charities, too. One of them I became involved with after meeting Kenneth Cole, a great honor because he is such an incredible humanitarian as well as clothing designer. Through him and Andrew Cuomo (the brother of Ken's wife, Maria), I signed on as a national board member for HELP USA, which provides housing and services

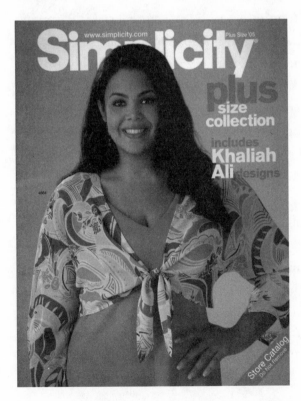

THIS CATALOG FOR SIMPLICITY SEWING PATTERNS CAME OUT IN THE SPRING OF 2005, ABOUT NINE MONTHS AFTER MY SURGERY. Courtesy Simplicity Patterns Company, Inc.

for the homeless, and as a spokesperson for HELP Philadelphia, a local chapter. Duties went from talking toy manufacturers into shipping toys to the kids in time for Christmas to story times with the youngsters and talking with the mothers in spiritual groups.

I also joined the National Center for Missing and Exploited Children, accepting an invitation to become that organization's national chairperson for its Minority Outreach Program—Hand in Hand with Children: Guiding and Protecting. They had me doing public service announcements on television, which I was happy to do, as I was actively losing weight.

Additionally, I became more involved with Culture Project, the New York group that puts on theatrical performances to give voice to disenfranchised members of society who would otherwise never be heard. (It was through Culture Project that I was invited to participate in the reading of the Constitution.) And, of course, I was still working with Wiggy at the Salvation Army's Soup's On! in Philadelphia.

I was socializing more, too. But as good as it all felt, it wasn't totally smooth sailing. A few months after the surgery, I found myself becoming incredibly emotional. I was very sensitive and cried easily. I remember one day I got in the car with Jacob and put on this Celine Dion tape called *Miracle*. It's about motherhood, and children, and birth. I always liked it, but that day, with every single song on the album, I cried my eyes out. Jacob just looked at me and said, "Mommy, what is wrong?" The tears were pouring out. I was so filled with emotion, so touched.

What I didn't realize at the time was that I was connecting with myself in a way I hadn't been able to before. It was like my senses were heightened. Previously, I had always eaten to block the process of "connect," but now I couldn't. Whatever I was feeling I had to let touch me. I was actually *coping* for the first time rather than running from my emotions, but I didn't have the word for it.

It wasn't always such a tender story. There were moments when I was in traffic, and you wouldn't have wanted to be in front of me. I had always been pretty docile, but I had a new kind of anger, or aggression, in me, that I had to deal with because I didn't have the mechanism of eating to defuse tension. I remember one incident, about four months out, when I had a really stressful moment with work. I was in a phone conference at home, and I hung up on someone. I felt like I was simply going to snap.

I went downstairs to pour a bowl of cereal. Then I got hysterical, realizing that option wasn't open to me. I had no choice, absolutely no choice, but to calm down, think through what had happened, and fix it the next day. It was extremely hard, that process of no longer isolating me from myself.

But I got better at it. I learned to calm myself with nonfood things. What other option did I have, since I wasn't hungry and couldn't fit much food down even if I were? I *had* to find new patterns, better patterns. So I'd surf the Net, read a book, even do a fifteen-minute exercise routine, anything to shake off the agitation that came with strong emotions, agitation that I had always shaken off with food. I would even follow all that advice that seems so facile but that really works—take a hot, luxurious bath or shower or clear away clutter.

I found that I could problem-solve better with my new distractions better than I ever could before. There's something about eating as a distraction that takes you away from problem solving. It's like a medication that dulls the senses. Food clouds things. Now my distractions were little breaks that I could return from refreshed. It was a happy discovery.

And then things got happier still. I had a second band tightening, several more weeks passed, and a week before Christmas I went to Drs. Fielding and Ren's office for a weigh-in and learned I had lost fifty pounds since my surgery. I was absolutely amazed at my success, but Drs. Fielding and Ren, while pleased for me, kept telling me I was not remarkable, that my weight loss was par for the course.

I was down to less than 250, because even though I had been 325 pounds at my highest, I had managed to lose some weight in one of my yo-yo cycles shortly before the operation. I had already been gaining it back close to the time of the surgery, but the band kept me from yo-yoing all the way back up, the way I always had my entire life.

The New Year brought new joys. One day I went to a Kenneth Cole fashion show, and when I entered the room, I sat front and center, and the hushed whisper was palpable. "Who's that girl? She's gorgeous. Is she a model?" It almost felt like an out-of-body experience. I knew it was me they were talking about, and I knew that at that point they still meant a plus-size model, but still, it was as if I were watching it while it was happening rather than experiencing it.

A couple of people came up to me. One of them was Carson Kressley, the blond guy with longish hair from *Queer Eye for the Straight Guy*, who said to me, "Honey, you are beautiful." That felt so good.

I, too, started looking at myself in a new way. Heavy people, myself included, neglect their bodies a lot. They literally avert their eyes from themselves; it becomes an unconscious habit. But I started to pay attention to my body. I remember thinking my skin was something people might be seeing more of, so I began using body oil. I had never been interested in examining myself before, in reminding myself what I looked like by touching myself. This was a whole new feeling.

I even started dating a little, nothing dramatic but getting my toes in the water, so to speak. The hardest part of it was realizing that so

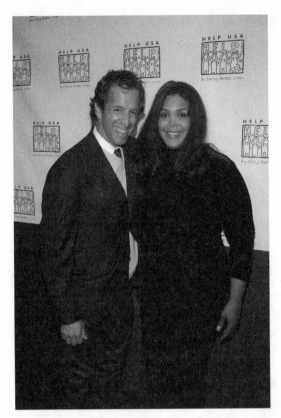

WITH KENNETH COLE AT AN EVENT FOR HELP USA. Courtesy Randy Brooke/WireImage.com

much of the dating ritual centers around food, around someone watching you eat. Then, too, how do you explain to someone you've just met, and who tells you how attractive you are, that you have a 325-pound past? (Not that I was anywhere near thin, but 235 or so is a lot thinner than 325.)

I decided to take the approach of being very up front with people. "Look, this is who I am, this is what I did." I felt if people couldn't deal with who I was up front, they weren't going to be able to deal with who I was in the long run. I don't know if that's the best tack to take for everyone, but it was the best one for me. It was all so complicated. I had never really dated in my life, and now here I was, out in the world getting a kind of attention that I wasn't used to, and it was a difficult balance between being my father's child, a single parent, and someone who'd undergone weight-loss surgery. I just didn't want to risk making things any more complicated or convoluted than they already felt.

While dating and working and losing weight and adjusting to the world's changing view of me, I continued working out. The difference was that I didn't sabotage my calorie burning in my workouts by going home and eating a peanut-butter-and-jelly sandwich on top of dinner, undoing my hour or two of hard effort at the gym in twenty minutes. Now the calories I burned through exercise stayed off. Half a protein bar or sometimes even just a few sips of water after an arduous sweat, and I was good to go.

It's a wonderful feeling, not having to have to wade through the self-hatred and self-castigation of "I blew it." You *can't* blow it. Even if you wanted to eat, say, an entire bag of Milano cookies, you could only fit down a couple. The band, properly tightened several times during the course of the first year after the surgery, takes care of everything. Snacking the old way becomes inconceivable—which is why with each passing day I loved the band more and more.

It was like a relationship. There's some getting used to each other, and I did hit some rough spots, like realizing I couldn't eat rubbery-textured foods like lobster or shrimp—they just wouldn't go down. I learned I couldn't eat red meat, either. By the time I chewed it enough to swallow it, it was too disgusting. Bread was out for the first several months, too—I would take too big a bite and it would clump up in a ball and not go past the band, which was hard because I really wanted it.

There were other learning curves as well. I would find myself hungrier two weeks before my period and able to eat more at that time. It scared me at first; I thought I'd start gaining weight back. But after several weigh-ins and band adjustments at the hospital, I realized that it's okay to go with true hunger. As long as you stop eating when your hunger feels relieved and don't go on to the point of starting to feel full (which can actually be a painful sensation with the band), you'll continue losing weight.

The long and the short of it is that over time, you hit a point where you and the band grow really comfortable with each other; you *enjoy* relying on it to keep your eating in check. I loved being able to go through a whole day confident that I'd be able to choose the foods I wanted to eat, eat the right amount of them, and lose weight. It was like a slice of heaven.

Before, it had been, "It's lunchtime, I'm busy, I'll just run through Burger King and get a cheeseburger, onion rings, and a shake." *Now,* if I felt hungry (and just because it was lunchtime didn't necessarily mean I was hungry), I might get a yogurt at a convenience store. By March of 2005, just seven months out, I was down to just about 220 pounds. I was eating 1,200 to 1,300 calories a day and feeling perfectly comfortable—no stomach rumblings, no light-headedness, no weakness.

Then something awful happened. Toward the middle of that month I started experiencing really bad acid reflux and tightness that went beyond the tightness I had been having with my adjustments. I felt like I was choking in my sleep. I couldn't get any food down and was losing weight too quickly, even for a gastric band patient. I hated to lie down because of how awful it made me feel, and I had black circles under my eyes from losing sleep.

Dr. Fielding felt I needed a break from the band, so he loosened it completely—drained out all the water—and I immediately felt some relief. I started to treat myself to foods I hadn't been having any of—Mediterranean pizza with feta cheese, olives, and spinach, lots of fruits and vegetables, things that just would not go down before, or not without a lot of effort.

Two weeks later I went back, had learned I gained about ten pounds, and got the band tightened again. "The party's over, doll," Dr. Fielding said. "Time for an adjustment."

But as soon as I got the tightening, I felt very sick again—choking, coughing, not being able to breathe properly. I couldn't even swallow my own saliva and even blacked out a couple of times. One night I went to the emergency room at Bryn Mawr Hospital, where they thought I might have had aspirational pneumonia but then ruled it out.

Ten days later, with no relief from the reflux, abdominal pain, or other symptoms despite being prescribed some medications that night in the emergency room, I was readmitted to NYU for Dr. Fielding to perform an investigative laparoscopy to find out, once and for all, what was wrong. It turned out I had a huge hiatal hernia—an out-pouching of the stomach several inches long that went above the band into the small, upper stomach pouch. That's what was causing all the problems, making things much, much tighter than they were sup-posed to be and acting as a food trap so that hardly anything I took in could make its way out of the herniated part of my stomach and into the lower stomach and on to the intestines.

What a huge relief to have the problem identified—and cor-rected. Shortly after the operation for the hernia (I needed only a one-night stay at the hospital), Dr. Fielding began a series of tighten-ing adjustments over several weeks, and I was back on track. Not that I ended up gaining any weight back during the ordeal. The weight I had gained in the two weeks after he drained out all the water came back off as soon as he retightened me the first time; I just couldn't get—or keep—anything down with the hernia in the way.

But now I was losing weight appropriately, without pain, and by the middle of May I was down to 199. Look, Ma, no diet pills!

That summer, just a few weeks after my one-year mark, I went to visit my father at his home in Michigan for the first time since the surgery. He had not seen me in more than 125 pounds, and he had not seen Jacob, now six years old, since he was a toddler.

The trip itself was unlike any long trip I had taken in years. I wasn't winded dragging luggage—and Jacob—through the airport. My joints didn't ache. My feet didn't swell.

I had been feeling better physically for quite a while—able to run up and down the stairs in my house, not sweating as much, not having to maneuver myself to get in and out of tight spaces. But the plane trip, in stark relief to so many other trips I had taken, really put into context just how far I had come. It was amazing to me to just be a regular passenger rather than feel like someone who was enduring a marathon. I loved, too, not having to worry about getting the seat belt across my lap—as well as not being the recipient of disapproving, or just plain gaping, stares as I made my way around a public space. That is, the new me was doing much better not just from the inside out but also from the outside in; the world was looking at me in a different way.

When we arrived, Jacob ran up to the door, and then there was my father on the other side of it, and my eyes welled up with tears. The two of them just looked at each other, and the first thing my father said to Jacob was "I love you." Jacob grabbed him and touched his face and said, "Pop Pop, I love you *more*." Then my father reached out and hugged him and just held him like that for a long, long time. It was full-faucet waterworks for me.

The visit was so wonderful. My father barely alluded to my weight, only sucking in his cheeks to show that he thought I looked skinny. I think he didn't want to hurt my feelings by telling me I looked better than ever, because his intention was *always* to make me feel beautiful, fat or thin. But my sister Hana, one of my father's other daughters, who was there for the visit and whom I'm very close to, told me afterward that he did ask her about the weight loss when I wasn't in the

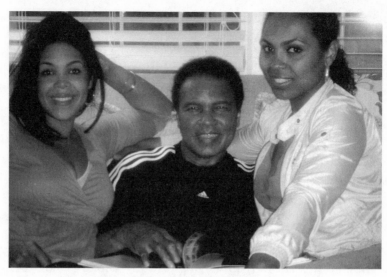

ME, MY FATHER, AND MY SISTER HANA A YEAR AFTER MY SURGERY.

room out of a sensitivity to what I might have felt was private. He wanted to make sure I had lost the weight in a healthy way and also that it hadn't happened as a result of illness.

I saw my father again three months later at the gala opening of the Muhammad Ali Center. ("Don't call it a museum," he said. "I'm not that old.") Housed in his hometown of Louisville, Kentucky, the center is an $80 million project, housed on six levels in ninety-three thousand square feet. Its goal is less to showcase artifacts and memorabilia of my father's life and more to serve as an international education and cultural center for promoting respect between people, hope, understanding, giving, and spirituality and to inspire both adults and children to be confident, to be as great as they can be.

It was a very, very proud night for me—and extremely exciting, as I was going to get to see my sisters on my father's side, many of whom I had not gotten together with for quite some time. Also, famous people from all walks of life were going to be there. *And* I didn't have to worry that I was going to look bad, mar the picture of my father with all of his beautiful daughters. I weighed 175—still somewhat overweight, but much, much thinner than obese, and even thinner still than morbidly obese.

It was a lot of fun to pick out a gown. For once I had an abundance of choices, not "thank God" if I came across even one thing that didn't make me look like a blimp wreck. I found what I wanted at Saks. It was a formfitting bias-cut black satin skirt that went to the ankles, with an Asian-inspired paisley print jacket—magenta, gold, and black—that had traditional Asian toggle buttons and a Nehru collar. The best part—I could tie a black satin ribbon around my waist.

The first people I saw when I arrived at the hotel where the family was staying were my identical twin sisters, Rasheeda and Jamilla. They looked more beautiful than ever. (Disney used their faces as inspiration in creating Pocahantas.)

Looking over swells of people who were there for the event, I rushed up to my room, where I had only a half hour to get ready because my flight had been delayed. But it didn't matter. I had much more confidence now, and it took me much less time to get ready to go into public.

I had been wearing my hair in a long braid—on purpose, because when I took out the braid, my hair looked wavy and I was able to just shake it out. I stared at myself in the mirror for a moment, allowing myself the pleasure of thinking, "You look good." I actually felt okay.

Downstairs, people were realizing who my sisters and I were because our father, to one degree or another, is marked on our faces. Then I was paid one of the highest compliments ever. A group of fifty or sixty kids starting chanting "Laila, Laila" as I walked by. I remember thinking, "Hell, I *must* look good if they think I'm Laila." I felt immensely proud of her. I felt like I come from a family of champions.

It truly was a family moment. There were five of my sisters with me, each as beautiful as the next, each a champion in her own way—and I actually fit in. I looked like I belonged.

It was soon time to go to the auditorium for the presentations and entertaining, but before that, when we were all together in a back room, someone called out, "We need everyone to clear the room except family. Clearance." A few moments later, in walked President Clinton. I couldn't have been more thrilled—or more flustered. It had been my plan to try to meet him at this event, and here the opportunity had fallen into my lap. I had always been a great admirer of his, and now that he was beginning his campaign to combat childhood obesity, my esteem for him had become even greater; we actually had personal common ground.

When he looked at me and shook my hand, I felt a blood rush but managed to muster, "Sir, this is a privilege. I'm proud to have this opportunity this evening." He was so gracious. I wanted to talk with him further about his initiative and perhaps could have pushed my way into getting more of his attention, but there were twenty-five people in a room that was ten by eight. I followed my rule about leaving such celebrity alone, although I did manage to get a picture with him later on that evening and talk to him for a moment with Dr. Fielding—he and Dr. Ren were my guests for the evening—about our desire to help children with weight problems so they didn't end up dieting casualties, like I did.

After the family's introductions to President Clinton, we were treated, with all the other guests, to a spectacular show. Singers included entertainers like James Taylor and Hootie & the Blowfish, and there were speeches by everyone from Bob Costas to Malcolm X's daughter, Attallah Shabazz, whose words brought tears to my eyes.

Then there was Jim Carrey. Everybody thinks of him as this comedic guy who makes goofy faces, but he was one of the most articulate and touching speakers I've ever heard, with a bearing like a true

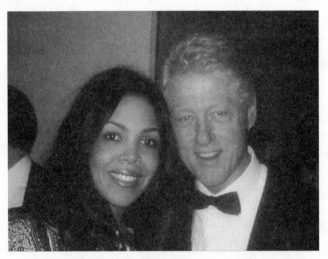

WITH BILL CLINTON AT THE OPENING OF THE MUHAMMAD ALI CENTER,
A LITTLE MORE THAN A YEAR AFTER MY SURGERY.

statesman (and incredible good looks, to boot). He talked about how he had it tough growing up but was always aware that he was born on my father's birthday, and that made him feel good things were in store for him. I'm not able to do his speech justice, but it was very affecting.

Jamilla had been dying to meet him, even before his speech, and after the festivities I was trying to figure out how I could arrange that,

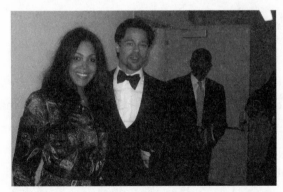

DR. FIELDING SNAPPED THIS PHOTO OF BRAD PITT AND ME AT THE OPENING OF
MY FATHER'S CENTER IN LOUISVILLE.

but as I was standing again in a back room, she came gliding in with him. I was so glad. Everyone was getting to make the introductions that were important to them.

Then, there in that room, I had a moment with Laila. Raised three thousand miles apart, under very different circumstances, we never really got to know each other that well, and there were some miscommunications because Jacqui Frazier-Lyde, whom Laila fought in the ring, is my dear friend. But Laila, who is four years my junior, pulled me aside and said, "Let me tell you something. You're my sister, you're my blood, and I love you. Anything you need, anything I have, is yours."

Tears were streaming down my face, and her eyes welled up, too. In that moment, my little sister was my big sister; her grace had gone through me and touched my heart.

But it was more than that. I had been fearing a harsh atmosphere that night between my sisters and me in general. When so many young women share a very famous father but have very different backgrounds and different relationships with that father, things can feel fractious, competitive. But they weren't. We all got along so well and felt so united; we felt whole with one another. So while it was obviously an evening all about my father, in a more personal way, it had been an evening about my sisters and me. We had formed a new constellation, and I left with my heart lighter.

||||||||||||||||||||||||||||||||||||||||||||||||||||||||||||||||||||||||||

A year is only a fraction of a person's life, but the year following a gastric banding packs in a lifetime's worth of changes. Khaliah's metamorphosis from scared, obese woman to healthy-weight and self-assured public figure says it all. Even the difference in the way she describes going to Philadelphia's Thirtieth Street Station right after she had the surgery and, a year later, taking her son through the airport to visit her father speaks volumes. Her tone about making her way through a public space was so much lighter once she had lost weight.

The change, of course, starts with the surgery itself.

When we get to a person's insides to perform a weight-loss operation, we know immediately whether the patient has been adhering to the prescribed liquid fast in the two weeks leading up to the operation. You can't hide it. Even in an extraordinarily obese person, a fourteen-day liquid diet will shrink the liver in both length and depth by two inches, so that instead of reaching to the belly button, it doesn't even go past the rib cage.

The reason it's so important to shrink the liver prior to the procedure is that the surgeon has to get past it—literally lift it up and to the side to reach the stomach. If the liver's too big and heavy, that makes it harder to do. It can get bruised if you push on it too hard, so it won't work that well for a while after the operation, not clearing toxins from the body as efficiently as it should.

We sometimes used to switch from laparoscopic surgery to regular surgery involving a large incision if the liver was too large to manipulate with laparoscopic instruments. Now we routinely stop the operation and close the person back up. We found it's not really easier to move the liver if you make a big cut—it's still in the way. Granted, in the thousands of bariatric surgeries we've performed, we've had to stop only a handful of operations because of a bloated liver. But why risk being one of the few who goes under anesthesia for nothing, leaving the operating room without the new lease on life you've finally decided to allow yourself?

When the banding surgery goes well, as Khaliah's fortunately did (her liver wasn't even really bloated; she strayed from the prescribed liquid plan less than she had built up in her mind), the patient generally feels some soreness rather than pain. In fact, most people who have undergone laparoscopic banding feel good enough to get out of bed and walk around a few hours after the surgery—which they should. That helps prevent blood clots and respiratory problems.

In the immediate postoperative phase, the majority of people experience a raw feeling in the upper stomach and a raw feeling when they swallow. It passes after a couple of weeks.

Sometimes, there's also an odd feeling in the left shoulder after eating, which also goes away in pretty short order. It's in large part referred pain. The stretching of the abdomen with carbon dioxide gas during the surgery also stretches the diaphragm, and the way the nerves are connected in that area of the body sends messages up to the shoulder. It's nothing to be concerned about, and it will in no way feel debilitating.

Most people go home the day after the surgery, although in some surgical centers, adjustable gastric banding is an outpatient procedure.

The first few days at home, the idea is to take it easy but not stay in bed. It's important to get up and walk around several times a day, taking deep breaths. Like walking through the hospital halls after surgery, it gets the blood circulating and helps prevent problems like blood clots and pneumonia, which can occur if you are too inactive following an operation. (Khaliah was right to walk to the mailbox and take slow strolls around her cul-de-sac.)

You are allowed to resume swallowing most medications you might be taking on the day you arrive home. Most people have no problems taking their pills after the surgery, although large tablets may need to be broken in half or crushed before swallowing.

A WORD ON PHYSICAL ACTIVITY

While we don't recommend staying perfectly still after the banding procedure, we also do not recommend that most band patients try to go full throttle into an exercise program early on. Many patients start out significantly heavier than Khaliah did, so any physical activity more strenuous than some very slow walking here and there could be very difficult—and harmful to the joints. A very heavy person's joints are already taxed by the pressure of the extra weight.

If someone feels she or he absolutely must exercise soon after the surgery, one safe option is swimming. The water carries the weight of the body and buoys the joints. But with swimming, particularly if it's in a public pool, there's often the psychological barrier of not wanting to be seen in a bathing suit.

The long and the short of it: gastric band patients should begin a regular exercise program after they've lost some weight and cleared it with their doctor. It's safer, and they'll be able to go at it with more confidence.

You will undoubtedly need less medication of almost any kind as time goes on. Weight loss resulting from gastric banding usually resolves or at least greatly reduces the effects of diabetes, high blood cholesterol, high blood pressure, certain forms of arthritis, and a host of other conditions.

Within a few days of arriving home, most people with a desk job can return to work. If you have a strenuous job or a job that requires heavy lifting, you may need to be off work or on light duty for a couple of weeks. (If you don't want anyone at work to

Illness	Resolved/Cured with Surgery(%)*	Improved(%)**
High blood pressure	58%	100%
High cholesterol	30%	68%
Diabetes	75%	92%
Degenerative arthritis (osteoarthritis)	52%	83%
Sleep apnea	94%	95%
Gastroesophageal reflux (heartburn)	79%	90%

*Illnesses resolved or cured in percentage of cases followed.

**Improvement in illnesses, but not complete cure, in percentage of cases followed.

know you've had weight-loss surgery, your surgeon can give you a generic doctor's note that does not specify the type of surgery you had. You are not required to disclose your personal medical history to your employer.)

The initial postoperative diet and reintroduction to solid foods varies somewhat from surgical practice to surgical practice, although there are usually at least a couple of weeks of just clear, low-calorie liquids. These include water, tea, Crystal Light, diet Snapple, Gatorade, broth, and, although not clear, a protein shake. It comes to some four hundred to eight hundred calories a day. (You can have coffee, too, even though it's not clear, but no cream—only skim or 1 percent milk.)

The liquid phase is crucial to your recovery. There are a few stitches holding the band in place that must not be disturbed until they heal, and if you go back to solid foods too soon and accidentally plug up the hole between the upper and lower stomach, you could vomit. That, in turn, might cause the stitches to tear, leading the band to shift position or slip, and then a second surgery is required. Also, the stomach itself needs time to heal right after the surgery, and solids are too much for it at that point.

A day's eating during the liquid phase might look something like this:

Breakfast: orange juice diluted with water, tea (with lemon) or coffee, protein shake.

Lunch: broth, protein shake, diet iced tea, clear fruit Popsicle.

Dinner: broth, Crystal Light, tea or coffee, clear fruit Popsicle, protein shake.

Snack: low-sugar juice; sugar-free Popsicle.

You will need to take very small sips at first. Too much or too fast can induce discomfort or pain and vomiting. You should also avoid drinking your beverages extremely cold, at least until you can sip them very gradually.

During this phase, about seven to ten days after the surgery, you will need to make your first postoperative visit to your surgeon to have your incisions checked and make sure everything's healing as it should.

After two weeks of thin liquids, you move on to the next phase of eating. In some surgical practices, that means starting on full liquids—everything from the first phase but now also non-fat milk, creamed vegetable soups, puddings, low-fat yogurt, pureed fruit, and instant breakfast or protein drinks.

At our practice at NYU, we go straight to what we call a mush or puree diet, which includes all the full liquids but also allows items such as soft-boiled or poached eggs, well-cooked oatmeal or creamed hot cereal with skim milk, a small mashed banana, cottage cheese, creamed vegetable soups, and applesauce. Some people are also able to tolerate canned or soft-cooked fruits and vegetables that have been pureed in a blender or fruit processor—good appliances to have on hand during this phase.

A day of eating during the mush phase might look like something like this:

Breakfast: ½ cup oatmeal with skim milk *or* a poached egg *or* a protein shake *or* a small mashed banana.

Lunch: ½ cup low-fat yogurt *or* ½ cup cottage cheese *or* 2 to 3 tablespoons tuna with a mild spread such as low-fat dressing *or* a hot vegetable such as ½ cup spinach, creamed with a bit of margarine and skim milk.

Dinner: ½ cup creamed vegetable soup *or* a small mashed (white or sweet) potato creamed with skim milk and a dot of margarine.

Snack: ½ cup low-calorie pudding *or* low-calorie frozen dessert.

This phase, too, lasts two weeks. Be very careful during this time not to overdo it with calories. For instance, you can make a soft casserole go down with added liquid, but if that liquid is gravy, you're going to be consuming more calories than are consistent with a healthful reducing regimen.

Don't forget to take extremely small bites during this phase and make sure all of your food is chewed extremely well, even though it is entering your mouth in an already-softened state. The softer the texture going down, the smaller your chance of experiencing stomach irritation, swelling, blockage, or vomiting.

Even more important is your rate of fork-to-mouth action. Spread out your bites. Put down your fork after swallowing, count to fifty, then pick up your fork for your next bite. The rate of swallowing predicts whether or not you will experience discomfort.

Do be sure to stay well hydrated through the day. Drink plenty of water, apart from what you might add to food.

Sometime during the mush phase, most banded patients lose the initial compulsion to keep feeling for the reservoir port that has been placed under their skin. It just becomes a part of you. (Men can usually feel it more easily than women because they have less external fat.)

In our practice, after two weeks in the mush phase—four weeks after the surgery—patients return gradually and cautiously to solid foods. (In some practices, solid foods don't reenter the picture until six weeks post-surgery.)

For better or worse, many patients also start to feel hunger, as Khaliah did. No hunger is felt until then because even though the band has not yet undergone its first tightening, or adjustment, the postoperative swelling in the stomach makes the band sort of snug on its own and impedes wanting to eat. Once the swelling settles, however, hunger returns. It frightens a lot of patients and makes them feel the band is not going to work. But the hunger is perfectly normal, and it's okay to regain some weight if you've been losing any before then.

That's because until the first adjustment, you are not in active weight loss. It is, rather, a time for healing and allowing the stomach to recover from the surgery and adapt to the presence of the band. If you do lose weight during that time, fine. But if you don't lose weight or lose some and then gain some back, that is fine, too. Be patient. It is infinitely more important prior to the first adjustment not to vomit than to lose weight. That, in fact, is much of the reason for the slow reintroduction to solid foods.

Go gingerly when first trying out solids.

- Start with very small portions.

- Cut all your food into small pieces.

- Eat slowly.

- Chew well.

- Put down your fork or spoon in between swallows. (It bears repeating.)

We cannot emphasize these instructions enough. You don't want to do anything to risk blocking the passageway between upper and lower stomach. It's like a blocked drain.

Add new foods one at a time. Then, if you have difficulty getting something down, it will be easier to identify the food that is causing you trouble.

You will find eating easier altogether if you mix your textures. For instance, take a bite of soft meat, and, after swallowing and waiting, take a bite of cracker or vegetable. All one food can bulk up and plug the stoma—the opening between the upper and lower stomach.

Keep in mind that texture is your friend because it provides clues to what you will be able to tolerate. Soft, flaky, tender, crumbly, and crunchy are band-friendly and tend to go down relatively easily. Chewy, rubbery, tough, and doughy are band-unfriendly. For that reason, most banders find they cannot eat bread. Remember when you were a kid and you pulled the crust off Wonder bread, then smushed it into a ball with your fist before you ate it? Well, that's what happens to bread when you try to eat it with a gastric band. It just forms a doughy ball right above your band, one that's not only too big to go down but that also blocks everything else from going down. (Crunchy bread sticks, crackers, and melba toast work much better.)

Whole chunks of meat like steaks and pork chops don't work for the majority of people with a band, either, at least not at first. Our teeth are not sharp enough to cut the meat into shreds small enough to go through the hole. What happens instead, even if you chew the meat a thousand times, is that it gets smashed up into a broad, pancakelike shape, ideally sized to block the band. Dr. Fielding has never been able to fit red meat through his band, although he and most other band patients are able to tolerate ground meat pretty well *if* it is well chewed.

Ground or not, it is better to make your first solid protein sources foods such as fish and beans. Fish is the best (and most healthful) choice for a band patient, particularly the flaky, moist white type. Salmon is also excellent.

Lean poultry cut up into extremely small pieces works for many, too, although it has to be without the skin, and it usually has to be dark meat instead of white—the dark meat is a bit juicier. (A lot of people vomit for the first time when they try a chicken sandwich on bread made with white meat. They test their band limits in the first couple of weeks and find that's one of them.)

Other foods that generally don't work with a gastric band, certainly not at first: shellfish like shrimp and lobster tail, which are rubbery; and leftovers, such as leftover fried rice, which can also get a rubbery kind of texture. There is no single food you should not try; it's just a good idea to be aware of the accumulated experience of those who have come before you.

Don't freak if, while you are experimenting with solids in those first two weeks of solid foods, you happen to vomit. Use it as a learning experience—to figure out what might have gone wrong. Did you eat the wrong food? Too much food? Too fast? Without very thorough chewing? Just about everyone vomits a few times. That's okay. You just want to make sure you minimize it. Fortunately, as Khaliah says, it doesn't feel like vomit coming up. It feels like the food, undigested. It's like when a baby regurgitates from suckling too fast, not like what happens when you have a nasty stomach bug.

SOLID FOODS TO EMPHASIZE IN THE FIRST SIX MONTHS

The following foods work very well for banders during their first six months of solids after the operation, both because they are nutritionally dense and easy to get down. Of course, these foods are good for you after the first six months, too.

- Fish, eggs, beans, ground meat
- Cheese
- Pasta (a band-friendly carbohydrate base to top with other foods, such as ground meat or flaked fish)
- Vegetables (and we don't mean french fries!)
- Fruits, particularly melon, papaya, strawberries, and mangoes. Stone fruits like peaches, apricots, and plums are okay if you remove the skin, as are apples. Citrus is more difficult to deal with because of the white pith between the skin and the fruit. That particular texture doesn't agree with the band.

The more slowly you eat solids, and the more carefully you choose your foods and chew them, the better off you will be when you get your first band adjustment, because band tightening makes it even harder to get away with eating too fast or eating the wrong things or chewing sloppily.

Most practices schedule the first adjustment for somewhere between four and eight weeks after the surgery. Adjustments take place on an outpatient basis and normally require only a few minutes. At the beginning, when there's still a lot of fat on your tummy, you may need to have your adjustments not in the surgeon's office but in the radiology department, where fluoroscopy—a moving X-ray—guides the surgeon to your reservoir port.

Right after the adjustment, it's a very good idea to have a drink of water. That's not a guarantee that the correct amount of fluid was injected, but it could potentially save you a second trip to the doctor. If the water does not go down, it's quite likely that you're too tight and need to have some fluid removed so the band will be a little looser.

For the first two days after a tightening, sip fluids slowly and reintroduce solid foods gradually over the course of a week. Initially, you're going to feel increased resistance when you first go to eat after a new adjustment, so you want to take extremely small bites, and take it slowly.

Sometimes, the stomach swells or becomes a bit irritated in the first day or two after an adjustment. The result is that solid foods become too uncomfortable to eat and you end up relying solely on liquids. That's okay because the effect is so short-lived. (But you should *always* be able to take in sufficient fluids. If you're spitting up saliva or regurgitating even liquid drunk slowly, the band is most likely too tight and necessitates an immediate call to your doctor. You never want to risk dehydration.)

At NYU, with the gastric band currently approved by the Food and Drug Administration, it's standard for everyone to be injected with 1 cc of fluid (a fifth of a teaspoon's worth) at the first band tightening. At the second adjustment, within a month or two, another cc of fluid is injected. About two months later at the third adjustment, most people get a half cc. After that it goes up in quarters, and even less than that sometimes once the fill level reaches 3 cc.

The average end-fill level for most people is anywhere from 2.75 to 3.5 cc, although some people need as many as 4 cc, and a few even need 4.5. The band can actually hold 5 cc, but we've rarely had anyone who needed that much. (There is a larger band that only recently came out that holds 11 cc, and the volumes are added a bit differently–3 cc at first, then 3 cc again, followed by 2 cc, 1 cc, and so on.)

Why do you need to keep getting the band readjusted? To go from zero to three all at once would simply be too hard on the body; you have to get there bit by bit. But also, as you lose fat, the band gets looser around the stomach, and you've got to maintain pressure to keep it working.

It usually takes about six or seven adjustments within the first year for a person to reach her or his own "sweet spot." After that, the adjustments are able to come less frequently–maybe once every three months in the second year and once every six months in the third year.

The band is at the right tightness if you're losing anywhere between one and three pounds a week. For instance, Khaliah, in the nineteen weeks between her August surgery and the week before Christmas, lost 50 pounds–just over 2.5 pounds a week. Her rate of weight loss went at a good, healthy clip. (It was not a remarkable clip for a gastric band recipient, as Khaliah thought in her amazement at her consistent weight loss. But *Khaliah* is remarkable!)

If you are losing more than a few pounds a week, your band may very well be too tight. Other signs that your band is too tight and that you should contact your surgeon, even without a scheduled appointment:

- You're unable to swallow your saliva.

- You have terrible chest pain after eating slowly and chewing thoroughly.

- You can't get down *any* solid food.

- You have frequent heartburn, belching, and regurgitation even after eating slowly and chewing thoroughly.

- You are experiencing symptoms that feel respiratory in nature—sore throat, wheezing, chronic coughing, or hoarseness.

Sometimes such symptoms are about something *causing* band tightness rather than band tightness in itself. Khaliah experienced many of these discomforts as a result of a hiatal hernia, which had the *effect* of making her band too tight.

It was her excess weight that led to the hernia in the first place. There was just too much pressure on her stomach, which is what caused a piece of it to push out and create its own extra pouch—the characterizing sign of a hernia.

But the outpouching didn't become apparent until after the banding, when the hernia ended up above the band and caused extreme, undesirable tightness. Where there should be one or two inches of stomach above the band, there were upward of three or four, causing excess acid pooling and other symptoms. Also, before the band surgery, the hernia was plugged with fat, so food couldn't get stuck in it. But after the surgery, during Khaliah's active weight loss, the hernia became unplugged and food was all too easily able to lodge in it, causing all kinds of uncomfortable sensations. Consider that she was able to get more food from her mouth into the upper part of her stomach as a result of the outpouching, but the food wasn't able to pass through the band into the lower stomach below the band.

We have found that roughly a third of our banding patients have hiatal hernias, and we now actively look for them and repair them at the time of the gastric band surgery. A band around the stomach should simply reduce hunger and restrict eating; it should not feel punishing. If it does, something is wrong.

In fact, if you have frequent vomiting that does not improve with your trying to eat more slowly or eat less, contact your surgeon. It could be anything from a band that was tightened too much to something more serious, such as band slippage. Do *not*

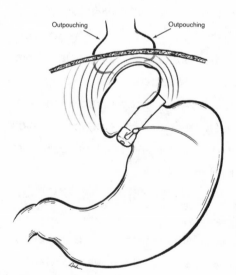

Outpouching   Outpouching

THE OUTPOUCHING ON EITHER SIDE OF THE STOMACH BY THE WALL OF THE DIAPHRAGM IS A HIATAL HERNIA, RELATIVELY COMMON IN OBESE PEOPLE. IT MUST BE CORRECTED IN ANYONE WITH A GASTRIC BAND.

simply switch to liquids or all soft foods in an attempt not to throw up. With just a few exceptions, you should be able to eat solid foods with a band and not have to pay a price.

The flip side of the too-tight coin, of course, is that sometimes the band is not tight enough, and the weight is not coming off. Signs that you might need a band tightening:

- You have not lost any weight for two to three weeks.

- Your appetite has increased.

- You are hungry fewer than four hours after eating a meal.

- You are able to eat more food during a meal.

- You are able to eat foods you were unable to eat before.

- You are snacking more often.

- You are *looking* for food.

Again, it's definitely time to call the surgeon's office, even if your scheduled appointment is not until some time in the future. The whole point of the surgery is that you are supposed to be able to lose weight without having to experience hunger all the time.

To help avoid emergency calls that might result from the fact that reactions to the band are not always identical, in our practice we urge everyone to come in once a month for the first year for a post-op consult with one of us or our nurses; a weight measure; and a possible band adjustment.

IT IS REALLY IMPORTANT NOT TO SKIP APPOINTMENTS FOR BAND ADJUSTMENTS. Not only can keeping appointments help guarantee that the band won't be too tight, our own research has also proven that people who have more than six visits during their first year after surgery lose more weight than patients who have fewer than six. It's not just the adjustments but the visits themselves. During visits, we provide reinforcement and counseling. Remember, the band is a tool; it is not, in and of itself, the solution. You have to work with it.

Because follow-up visits and frequent band adjustments are so important, our fee for an adjustment is $100. Some other practices charge as much as $300 to $400, especially on the coasts. Granted, most insurance companies pay for adjustments. But insurance often doesn't cover the entire cost of the adjustment—a major impediment to patients coming back as often as they need to and losing weight as quickly as the band can let them.

What is a band patient's general diet like once the initial adjustments have taken place and life really starts getting back to normal? It's like the same reasonable, balanced diet you've been on a hundred times before: about 1,000 to 1,200 calories a day for women, 1,200 to 1,500 for men. In fact, many of our patients attend Weight Watchers as a guide to eating sensibly: two servings a day from the dairy group, four to six ounces of protein-rich food, two to three servings of vegetables, one to two pieces of fruit, three to four starches, and very little in the way of added butter, margarine, dressings, or oil. The difference is that you don't walk around starving in order to lose the weight. Life feels comfortable, *normal*.

Here are some tips for maximizing the band's effect.

1. Stop eating at the first hint of fullness. Don't eat until you are signaled to stop by chest pain, burping, hiccuping or other discomfort, or throwing up. You can always

eat more later, if you are still hungry. But chances are you won't be. If you stop eating and busy yourself with something else, you will forget about food until your body says it's truly time to eat again.

2. Go with the flow. That is, you will be reminded that the band is inside you when you eat too fast, eat too much, have not chewed properly, or have eaten something that is too tough and cannot pass. It will feel like chest pain, and it will be relieved by waiting until the food passes through or you regurgitate it. To avoid unpleasant sensations, always take it slowly, and don't overeat.

3. Drink six to eight glasses of water a day. The water will keep your pouch busy.

4. Drink liquids before, not during, meals. Drinking after you have already taken bites will cause the food to flush through the small upper pouch more easily, making you hungrier for more.

5. Don't drink any liquids with calories other than two glasses of skim milk a day and up to two alcoholic beverages (one if you're a woman). Liquids pass through the pouch very quickly and will not make you feel full, no matter how many calories they have.

6. In the main, go for denser, less processed foods such as fresh fish and meats, fruits, vegetables, and beans. They are relatively difficult to eat—you have to slow down, take smaller bites, and chew more—so they will make you feel more satisfied than softer, processed foods that

pass through the band all too easily. Of course, they're also better for you than foods with a high concentration of calories and little nutrition value—all the more important since you need to get all your vitamins and minerals from much less food than you've been used to. It doesn't mean you can never eat a chocolate chip cookie or have a half cup of ice cream or a piece of chocolate. It just means that, as always, such treats should be occasional rather than constants in your life. The mainstay should be foods that swim, fly, or grow in the ground. (Don't worry. The lack of hunger takes care of most of the cravings.)

7. Don't graze throughout the day, which makes it easier to get more food down in small increments. Instead, plan up to three meals a day and up to two snacks. A snack (or even a meal) may be a half cup of low-fat yogurt, a protein bar, or two or three crackers with a little cheese. You may find you can't eat two snacks daily or three meals. That's okay. Go with your hunger, or rather, your lack of hunger. Each day will differ in terms of your hunger and the amount of food you need to satisfy it.

8. With your physician's approval, once you've lost a significant amount of weight ("significant" will be different for different people), engage in regular physical activity. After gastric banding, exercise is just as important as you've always heard it was. It also has the potential to blunt sharp rises and falls in blood sugar that contribute to hunger, and it's a good antidote to not being able to turn to food all the time as an outlet for emotions. How you choose to move your ever-thinner body doesn't have to be overly taxing. You can even do all those things that

are always listed in magazine articles but that few people take advantage of: park away from the mall or supermarket entrance, take the stairs instead of the elevator, walk for any errand that's under a mile, and so on. Tucking in bits of activity here and there really does add up to a beneficial effect on your body.

9. Join a support group. This might be the most important advice of all. Getting a gastric band is no small thing. There's a lot of adjusting to do physically, and a lot of psychological reckoning that goes on as well. Talking it all out with other people going through what you're going through can be tremendously relieving as well as encouraging.

It's great if your surgeon heads or initiates a support group, because everyone in it will be following the same instructions. It's better still if everyone in the group has had the same type of weight-loss surgery rather than if some have gone through banding and others have had gastric bypass, which entails a whole different set of lifestyle recommendations and a somewhat different mind-set, too. (Gastric bypass is like a supertight gastric band for one year, with no adjustments during or after.) When everyone's in the same boat, they can share not only experiences, feelings, and problems but solutions, too.

We head an ever-growing support group for our NYU patients. Everything gets discussed. For instance, Khaliah noted that she can eat more in the two weeks leading up to her period. In a support group, women will find that others have the same experience, and the same fear that the band is not working well enough. But Dr. Ren has explained that the force with which the esophagus propels food into the stomach is dependent, in part, on hormone concentrations, and in the second half of the month, hormones work to push down more food.

So what you might learn in a support group is that it's okay to feel a little hungrier before your period and to eat a little more, as long as you don't force food down and end up regurgitating. Conversely, you may learn that you're apt to feel much less hungry after your period, and that if you eat despite not being hungry, you could end up more uncomfortable. It's a way of helping women stay in touch with their bodies rather than get nervous that their bodies are betraying them. If you stop eating as soon as you don't feel hungry anymore, neither your body nor your band will work against you.

People also talk in their support groups about getting used to eating after band adjustments, about how they might have to wait ten seconds between bites of scrambled eggs but a whole minute between bites of a salad, which goes through the band more slowly. Those stories are validating, because it makes others with the band realize they're not alone in their sensations.

Food grief gets discussed, too. Khaliah experienced a little of it, not being able to eat the Italian meal she prepared for her family, and so on. But as the band gets tightened, patients really do lose the urge to eat, even the things they love. Khaliah was one of them. As you saw, she talked about missing eating the way she used to eat shortly after her surgery, but not as the months passed.

Only about 5 to 10 percent of banders end up with persistent food grief, continuing to want foods they love but are no longer physiologically hungry for. We are usually able to "gentle" such people through it, but if not, it might be appropriate to bring, say, a spouse or significant other to a tightening appointment. That way, the surgeon can have a substantive talk about relationships and food in the home, and in some cases recommend therapy so that emotional issues getting in the way of successful use of the band can be addressed by a mental health professional.

Another topic that might come up during a support group meeting is the fact that if you're nervous, you can't swallow as well. Of course, many people are nervous when they're new to the band and out eating with other people—the last instance in which they want to end up needing to regurgitate. So we talk about staying calm and how the band will work for you if you let it.

Then, too, there are holiday dinners and such, where most people with gastric bands start out perfectly ready and willing not to overeat but then get told by family members that they're not eating enough. So, falling into old family patterns, 10 to 15 percent of them eat more than they really want in order to comply and then throw up, only to be told by their loved ones, "See, the band doesn't work. Give it up."

There are two ways to deal with that problem. One is to refuse to let relatives be saboteurs, remaining polite but firm, even getting up from the table or missing a holiday get-together, if necessary. The other is to take a band break with a total loosening before a cherished family tradition such as Christmas dinner or a Passover seder. The thing is, if you do take a break, you have to get retightened once the holiday's over. Khaliah has seen how quickly you can gain weight back once the band is loosened, and so has Dr. Fielding. During a two-week vacation at Christmas one year, he put on sixteen pounds!

Band breaks are not the big talk at meetings, however. What gets discussed more than anything in the support groups—more than loosenings and family meals and saboteurs and food grief—are the simple nuts and bolts of really learning how to live with a gastric band, how to eat with it. For instance, some people just don't "get" volume, and the fact that the typical volume for a meal with a tightened band might be as little as a half cup of food. They say they eat like birds, but the birds might be vultures or eagles rather than hummingbirds. So they end up regurgitating, or grazing throughout the day and then not losing weight, or not losing significant weight.

Thus, a lot of what we go over is the art of eating small portions, slowly. We talk about the fact that the band provides *signals* to stop eating, like hiccuping and pain, and that you should not try to eat through the pain.

We don't just do it lip service. We dine with our patients to demonstrate eating with a band (and, as far as we know, we are the only surgeons who do).

For instance, one month Dr. Fielding took about twenty of his patients to an Italian restaurant for one of his "Learn to Eat with George" evenings. (September is Italian month.) They all started out eating as if they didn't have the band—too quickly, and without thorough chewing. It came from social pressure. Even around other band recipients, people often try to eat the way they always have so they can camouflage the fact that they have an apparatus inside their bodies. But it doesn't work.

Dr. Fielding finally said, "Everyone, stop." He showed them, literally, "This is how fast you eat. This is when you put your knife and fork down. This is when you take a sip of wine. This is when you have conversation. *This* is when you take another bite."

Seeing these behaviors in person makes a lightbulb go off in people's heads. They realize that instead of making you a social pariah, eating with a gastric band makes you a fine diner, elegant. And when you're done, you're done. No need to eat more once you're no longer hungry, no matter how much food is left on your plate.

Dr. Fielding and Dr. Ren have "taught" gastric band eating

not only in an Italian establishment but also in a French bistro, a kosher restaurant, and a sushi bar. (Sushi's easy. The rice is perfectly textured for making it through the band without difficulty.)

The eating practicums have become so popular for our patients that we have even gone on a dinner cruise around New York Harbor in order to accommodate more people. It's an incredible way of teaching everyone, even if they start out looking like linebackers, that they need to adjust to eating according to their hunger, which is to say they need to adjust to eating like a petite, size-six woman.

The eating sessions raise confidence. Think about it. One of the major reasons anyone has gastric banding surgery in the first place is to live a normal life with normal social activities, and eating with friends in a convivial social setting is part of that life. Now people who have undergone banding surgery get to have this rather than walk into eating establishments mortified that anyone who looks at them will immediately think they have no right to be enjoying their food.

Here's the eating lesson in a nutshell:

1. Relax. Eating with people is more about the company than the food, anyway. And, as we said before, if you keep relaxed, the food will go down more easily and you won't be excusing yourself to run to the bathroom to get rid of what won't pass through the band. (People who feel nervous tend to eat faster, which can cause chest pain and regurgitation with the band.)

2. When you go out, forget the rule about not drinking water or other beverages with your meal, just for that evening.

3. Have a settling drink, if you enjoy social drinking— sherry, champagne, wine, whiskey, a martini, or whatever other alcoholic beverage you like (except a mixed drink unless you use diet mixers, because fancy mixed drinks like Cosmopolitans are typically loaded with calories). Up to one drink a day for women, two for men, helps keep the esophagus from having spasms.

4. Don't eat any bread. None at all! It will get stuck.

5. Have soup as an appetizer if you see a soup on the menu that you happen to like. Other good appetizer choices: chopped salad, sashimi, creamy risotto. Avoid shrimp and calamari, as well as nuts.

6. Avoid all solid cuts of red meat, especially steak. Even in a steak house, have the salmon or tuna.

7. Avoid anything with cold chicken, turkey, or duck. Dark portions of these birds are okay served hot, *as long as they are moist.* If the bird is a bit dry and you eat it, you will be excusing yourself from the table to locate the nearest bathroom.

8. Don't sit there and cut your food into microscopic pieces and chew it fifty times. Nobody else does. Instead, have a little bit, chat, then have a sip of wine, smile, push the food around awhile, then have a little more. As Khaliah mentioned, nobody even really notices how much you're eating if you *act* like you're eating. Just play it cool, and take your time. It'll make you look like a sophisticated Parisian, enjoying every bite rather than shoveling it down.

9. If you think something might be stuck, don't leap to your feet and run as fast as you can to the bathroom. You are not going to vomit there and then. Instead, just ride it out for a while. Try to sit up straight, and breathe normally. (Again, the band always acts tighter when you're stressed.) Then, if it's no better, casually excuse yourself. People do go to the bathroom.

10. Pass on dessert. You have to watch calories. Not that you will have eaten very many. There's no way you're going to be digging into much of what's put in front of you with a properly tightened band. But even two bites of flourless chocolate cake can contain between fifty and one hundred calories. Over time, those little indiscretions add up. Let your lack of hunger be your guide.

We don't mean to make it sound difficult; it's not. It just takes a little getting used to. And it gets easier as you gain confidence; continue to lose weight without hunger; and find you have more energy and are able to do chores or play with children and not lose your breath.

Gradually replacing feelings of self-consciousness and shame with confidence and a sense of self-efficacy feels good, too, as does increased social acceptance and newly opened doors for better work opportunities, friendships, and intimate relationships. It is not infrequent for gastric banding patients who were on welfare to find employment or for people who were single to marry.

We are not trying to say that gastric banding is a magic wand that cures all of life's ills, because it isn't. But it *is* something you can use to achieve a healthier and fuller life, because it allows you to get a handle on proper diet and exercise without suffering.

And it does have its magic-wand qualities. As Dr. Fielding can attest, actually looking forward to getting glimpses of yourself in the mirror doesn't hurt. It's also uplifting, as Khaliah said, to have an abundance of choices that look good on you when you go clothes shopping rather than having to settle for the drab-colored "tent" or suit from the "portly" section.

Finally, it feels good not to have to huff and puff just to do things that other people take for granted, like walk quickly to make a meeting on time, pull wet laundry out of a washing machine, or enjoy a day of sightseeing. These may sound like relatively small details, but they're life altering.

8

THE COLOR LINE, THICK AND THIN

At Madison Avenue ad agencies, in universities, and at civil rights organizations, marketers, scholars, and advocates for racial equality are debating whether the image of the large, sassy, brassy, black woman who doesn't take any guff is an acceptable or offensive characterization. Last year, while they were arguing the merits of such figures as the spokeswoman in the Pine-Sol ad, my friend Kim, a very large black woman herself, died suddenly of a massive heart attack.

Kim was not bold and brassy. Thirty-seven years old, she was a quiet woman, the manager of a successful real estate agency, and a single mother who had finally saved up enough money for her gastric banding operation after having been denied coverage by her health insurer. But instead of going for her surgical consult as she had planned, she was lying in a box, leaving behind two children, ages fifteen and twelve.

I didn't feel bold and brassy when I was an overweight woman "of color," either. I felt sad and insecure—and vulnerable. Kim paid the ultimate price of vulnerability, of course. But obesity renders you vulnerable in all kinds of ways, every day of your life, no matter what color you are (and we all have a color, so "of color" doesn't really make any sense).

Not only are you subject to the rudeness and downright nastiness of people who feel it's okay to let you know they disapprove of your body, you also can't go about your normal, everyday business without becoming winded or without your joints aching. You can't sit down on a crowded bus or subway train because the amount of room available on the one empty seat isn't enough to keep the person on either side of you from being annoyed that you dared to try to squeeze yourself in. But most importantly, you can't escape the very real risk for debilitating conditions that obesity levies: diabetes, high blood pressure, kidney problems, arthritis, sleep apnea, heart disease, certain cancers, respiratory problems, acid reflux, urinary incontinence, skin infections, infertility, and the list goes on. That is, vulnerability is obesity's middle name, even though large people are often thought of not as weak but as strong, as being able to "stand up to" things.

African American women are the most apt to be obese. I use the term *African American*—and *black*—somewhat loosely because, as the immediate past chair of the Department of African and African American Studies at Harvard, Henry Louis Gates Jr., pointed out in a fascinating PBS special, many people perceived to be of strictly African ancestry have a significant amount of genetic material from other continents. That is, someone might be 100 percent black *culturally* and identify strictly as an African American, but her DNA tells another story. In fact, African Americans, on average, are 20 percent European. Quincy Jones is 34 percent European, Professor Gates noted, while Whoopi Goldberg is 8 percent European. My own mix is considerable, as I am Irish, Portuguese, Japanese, Native American, Jewish, slave black, and British. (Family legend says that we are descendants of Henry Clay, speaker of the House decades before the Civil War. That's where the "Clay" in Cassius Clay comes from.)

Imperfections in classifying people based on their complexions rather than their DNA notwithstanding, here are some stats on the obesity-related differences between so-called African Americans and European Americans, culled by Drs. Fielding and Ren from the most recent government tallies available. (There are no statistics specifically for Haitian Americans and other black Americans whose ancestors were not engulfed in the U.S. slave experience. Everyone's lumped together as "black" or "white.")

Among white men, 29 percent are obese; among black men, 28 percent, which makes it pretty much a wash for males. But the numbers diverge greatly for women. About 31 percent of white women are obese, compared to a full 50 percent of black women.

When it comes to what is known as class-three obesity—morbid, or extreme, obesity defined as a body mass index higher than forty (someone who is five feet nine inches and weighs more than 270)—the discrepancy between white and black women is even greater, at least by one method of measuring. Five percent of white women are extremely obese, compared with 15 percent of black women—*a threefold difference.* And the proportion of extremely obese black women is rising much faster, more precipitously, than the proportion of extremely obese white women.

There are no doubt numerous reasons for the difference in obesity rates between white and black women, among them, lack of access in black urban neighborhoods to large, well-stocked supermarkets with affordable fresh fruits and vegetables and lean meats and whole grains. People in the inner city frequently must resort to convenience-store fare, which is expensive, fatty, caloric, and lacking in nutrients.

But there is also a cultural reason for the difference. Largeness, or thickness, in a woman is more acceptable, and often even more desirable, in the African American community at large. Generalizations are always dangerous, because you can always find black men who like skinny women and white men who prefer plump ones. But it's fair to say that on the whole, extra pounds on a black woman do not turn black people off.

Research has highlighted the point. When scientists at Yale analyzed a number of papers on people's concepts of obesity, the studies consistently showed that a larger body size is more socially acceptable, and more desirable, to black women and men than to whites. But you don't need research to prove it.

Think of the sitcom *My Wife and Kids,* with Damon Wayans. The wife, played by Tisha Campbell-Martin, is by no means obese, or even overweight, but she is certainly full-figured. You'd never find a wife or other female costar on a sitcom peopled by European Americans with that much behind or belly. (Think of Patricia Heaton on *Everybody Loves Raymond* or the actresses on *Friends.*)

An African American acquaintance of mine, Nick, perhaps puts it best when he says, "I like women thick. I don't really like skinny women. If there's some meat on the bones, it's good for me. I'd be okay with a woman who was two hundred pounds."

Mo'Nique, the size twenty-two star of UPN's *The Parkers* and author of *Skinny Women Are Evil,* goes so far as to celebrate fatness on women, saying that F.A.T. stands for "fabulous and thick" and relating how she told the producers of her show that just because her character was fat, she could not be portrayed wearing muumuus and sitting around the house all day. She would have to go out on dates, have adventures, boyfriends. (The producers complied, which was part of what made the show so engaging.) Mo'Nique has even staged full-figured beauty pageants on television to get across the idea not only that fat women deserve respect but that they are beautiful because "beauty comes in more than a size two."

I agree. It's hard for me personally because, not having grown up among mainly people who identify as black but, rather, in a multi-racial tableau that included many members of my family as well as friends, teachers, and others of European stock, I was introduced early on to the notion that "thin" and "beautiful" go together while "heavy" and "beautiful" do not. In fact, there are times when I'm disappointed about not having come through my surgery a stick and must remind myself, for instance, that I've inherited my father's big, strong calves; that the fact that I will never be perceived as petite doesn't make me "less than."

Also, while many people of darker color in my orbit happen not to be bothered by the stereotypical image of the large, feisty black woman, I tend to find its pervasiveness somewhat offensive. It's not just because it obfuscates the fact that there are large black women who are sad, who are meek, who are all kinds of things that are not bold and brassy. To me it also seems like some kind of flip-side-of-the-same-coin hand-me-down from Scarlett O'Hara's mammy in *Gone with the Wind*—a large woman who wasn't afraid to speak her mind but who "knew her place." Thus, those media images don't help me appreciate largeness among women in the black culture. They make it seem to me, instead, that outsize black women are somehow being relegated to the outskirts of the larger culture, interesting and amusing but bit players at the edges of the real action precisely because of their consistent rendering as two-dimensional "types" rather than as more fully realized characters.

Still, whether the stereotyping bothers you or not, all women, no matter what their size, do deserve to be considered beautiful, desirable, sexy, worthy, and everything else that defines a person you want to have in your life.

But the rub, ultimately, is not in the way the extra pounds make a large African American woman look. It's in how her weight plays out on her body. And many obesity-related diseases are found in higher rates among various members of racial-ethnic minorities than among whites. These include diabetes, hypertension, cancer, and heart disease. Here, again, are some stats.

Diabetes has been reported to occur at a rate of anywhere between 16 and 26 percent of black Americans ages forty-five to seventy-four, compared with only 12 percent in whites the same age. What's more, African Americans with diabetes are more likely to develop complications from the disease—and experience greater disability from those complications—than their European American counterparts.

How much that has to do with the difference in blacks' access to health care and how much with a genetic predisposition to diabetes is the subject of a book in itself. Research has suggested that many African Americans and recent African immigrants to the United States have a gene that increases their chances of getting the disease, and even a genetic propensity to put on weight. But the fact is that compared to their European American counterparts, African Americans with diabetes experience higher rates of diabetes fallout in the form of blindness, kidney failure, and lower-limb amputations. Black women, in fact, are three times as likely as white women to become blind from diabetes, while black men are 30 percent more likely to go blind than white men.

When it comes to lower-leg amputations resulting from diabetes complications, the higher rate for black Americans varies, depending on which research paper you look at. One study of hospital discharge figures showed that the amputation rate for African Americans with diabetes was 19 percent higher than for whites. In another study that took place in California, blacks were 72 percent more likely to have diabetes-related amputations than whites.

Obesity is presumed to have played at least some role, and along with affecting the prevalence of diabetes and its complications, it appears to contribute to the higher risk for pancreatic cancer among black Americans than among whites, particularly for women. In addition, 43 percent of blacks have cardiovascular disease, according to the American Heart Association, as opposed to just 33 percent of whites.

Obesity in African Americans is also a contributing factor in their high prevalence of hypertension, which hits blacks earlier in life and takes a more severe course than in whites. Hypertension, in fact, is an even greater contributor to kidney failure in blacks than diabetes. (Once you reach end-stage kidney failure, you have to go on dialysis and hope for a kidney transplant.)

Then, of course, there are the death rates. Severely obese black women twenty to thirty years old can expect to lose up to five years of their lives; severely obese black men, up to *twenty* years. According to research conducted at the University of Alabama, obesity begins to consistently steal years from black men when they reach a body mass index of thirty-two or thirty-three (about 240 pounds on someone six feet tall, and well *below* the weight at which a man would be considered a candidate for obesity surgery). Women appear to begin to lose years consistently when their BMI reaches thirty-seven to thirty-eight (about 225 pounds on someone five feet five inches).

Much of what it comes down to is that while very large black women, and the men in their lives, might be fine with how they look, all the excess weight simply is not good for them. It's not a matter of playing into a white idea of what beautiful is; it's a matter of life and death.

Fortunately, as I've learned from Drs. Fielding and Ren and some of their patients I've spoken with, it's possible to have it both ways.

Undergoing gastric banding doesn't have to come with the goal of becoming skinny, or even just plain thin. It can come with the goal simply of losing enough weight to resolve various obesity-related health problems—and that's often considerably less weight loss than people might think.

One young African American woman who came to them for a band, Mary, needed relief from horrible back pain. She was suffering so much that she would literally have to crawl into her orthopedist's office for a steroid injection to relieve the agony. It was too difficult to walk, or even bend over. The orthopedist told her that if she did not lose weight, her knees were going to give out in a few years.

Mary, five feet nine inches and 270 pounds, had not been at all worried about attracting men at her weight, and she did not have issues with her self-esteem. It was simply a matter of being able to use her body.

Initially, she felt disappointed in herself that she couldn't lose weight on her own, but today, four years after her banding procedure, that is not what concerns her. What matters now is that she is down to two hundred pounds and completely pain-free. And she has absolutely no intention of losing any more weight. "I recently went to a wedding," she said, "where people who hadn't seen me in a while told me I look good, but don't get any smaller."

It was a similar story for another of Dr. Fielding and Ren's patients, Shawna. At the age of twenty-nine, she was five feet seven inches and 260 pounds, having awful problems with her knees and back troubles, too. "There was no self-image issue," she says. "My family and friends always made me feel comfortable, and I did not have trouble getting dates. The surgery was for my pain."

Today, two years out, Shawna is down to a curvy 170 pounds, where she's perfectly comfortable, and pain-free. "I feel better" all around, she says. "I can run up a lot of stairs without sweating or feeling like I'm out of breath. It's also easier to carry things. And I can get a seat on the bus or train where I wouldn't have tried to sit down before. If it's a rush-hour train, I can push in without people trying to make me feel funny. Those things are priceless to me.

"You don't get a band because, 'Now, I'll be beautiful,'" Shawna adds. "You were beautiful before. You get it because the weight is wearing and tearing on your body."

Drs. Fielding and Ren say Shawna's attitude has been their experience in general. "With white women," Dr. Ren says, "the emphasis is more on wanting to look a certain way. Yes, they want to resolve health problems, but they often have a goal weight in mind and a goal for size, which is often an eight.

"The black women who come in, when I ask them their expectations for after the surgery, tend not to have a goal weight. They've never been pressured to be thin, so they don't have that uppermost in their minds. They have their medical concerns on their minds. They might tell me, 'Well, the chart says I should weigh one-forty.' And when I ask them what size they imagine themselves being, they'll say a ten, twelve, fourteen.

"Many make clear that they don't want to lose *too much* weight. They're not looking to become model thin but, rather, retain some curve and substance while getting healthier. Tyra Banks is not their ideal body type. She's not their husbands', either. The men will often say that they don't want their wives getting too skinny, which is not something you tend to hear from the white spouses.

"There *is* overlap, of course. *All* the women who come in want to shop at regular clothing stores. They want to get out of Lane Bryant. Those who have never been thin would also like to weigh less than two-hundred. The two-hundred mark is a big milestone in both races. But the women of African ancestry are not as concerned about the number on the scale per se. It's more an issue of their needing to be healthier."

Unfortunately, no more than 5 percent of the people who come to Drs. Fielding and Ren for bariatric surgery are African American, even though blacks make up 14 percent of the population. They are not availing themselves of the band.

The good news is that those who do come—even if their goal is not to slim down to anywhere near model thin—are just as likely to get rid of their health problems as those of European descent, and therefore just as likely not to have their lives cut short prematurely because of obesity. Drs. Fielding and Ren just quantified it in a three-year study that they recently presented at the annual meeting of the American Society for Bariatric Surgery. When they matched about sixty European American patients with some sixty African American patients for age, gender, and pre-op body mass index, they found that about two-thirds to three-quarters of the those in both groups had major improvements in or complete resolution of several major weight-related conditions, which included diabetes, hypertension, obstructive sleep apnea, high blood cholesterol, and high tryglycerides.

Yes, the African Americans did lose less weight—an average of 41 percent of their excess poundage after three years of follow-up as opposed to 52 percent of extra pounds for the European Americans. But the smaller weight loss did not impact the improvements in their health. In fact, for every single condition except high cholesterol, there was a trend toward more improvement for the blacks (with complete resolution for black patients of both diabetes and high triglycerides, risk factors for heart disease).

It's hard to say if the reason the blacks lost less weight was completely about cultural differences in attitude toward body thickness. While African Americans, particularly women, may not be as encouraged by their families and social circles as European Americans to lose the extra weight since it does not carry the same stigma, there could be a biological component as well. Dr. Ren says one idea that gets floated around has to do with differences in body composition. At least some research suggests that African Americans are more muscularly dense than European Americans. And muscle weighs more than fat, so when you have weight-loss surgery and lose fat, the greater proportion of muscle remaining on the black patients could translate into somewhat less weight loss.

Whatever the reason for the difference, it's important to note that not all weight-loss surgeons have had Dr. Fielding and Ren's experience. One doctor who spoke at their annual conference said he did *not* find differences in weight loss between whites and blacks after their bariatric surgeries. In other words, as Drs. Fielding and Ren would be the first to say, there are unknowns and variables affecting the rate of weight loss that have yet to be determined.

But that's not really the relevant point. What's relevant is that whoever you are, you can lose enough weight with a stomach band to greatly improve your health without losing so much that you wouldn't be perceived as looking good to your peers and loved ones.

Shawna makes the point most succinctly when she says, "You don't have to be nervous about losing too much weight. With the band, you have the control factor." That is, *you* decide how tight the band is going to be, and therefore, you can slow, and stop, your rate of weight loss at any point—either when your health problems have dissipated or, going further, when you're closer to (or at) a more slender standard for looking good.

If only my friend Kim had gotten to make that decision.

9

A CALL TO ARMS

My highest weight was 268. When I got the band, I was 248. My low weight after the operation was 135. I now hover around 150.

The band saved my life. I never would have survived my stroke at the high weight, what with all the procedures they had to perform on me. Or I would have been a stroke victim in a wheelchair, drooling.

That's my mother talking. By the time she was forty-eight, she had ballooned into the upper two hundreds, in part because the steroids she has to take to help keep her lupus in check make it extremely difficult not to overeat. It turns a very serious situation more serious still, because my mother has to deal with chronic complications from lupus, and all the extra weight (she's five feet three inches) makes treatment that much more difficult.

She had wanted bariatric surgery for years and was even willing to go for gastric bypass, which I talked her out by begging and pleading because I didn't want her to take that risk. But two months after my surgery, she was in the OR with Dr. Fielding, getting her own band.

She recovered even more quickly than I did, getting up sooner and walking faster through the hospital halls. I think that because she has lived with lupus most of her life and has dealt with so much pain, what registers as pain or soreness in others doesn't faze her.

She couldn't have gotten her surgery at a more propitious time. About a year later, her lupus attacked her brain, causing inflammation there and a series of transient ischemic attacks, or TIAs, which are tiny strokes. She was in the hospital for quite a while, having to receive a lot of medical intervention that, with a very large body, she might not have been able to withstand. The band truly did save her life.

My mother is one of only a number of people in my life who went and got a gastric band because of my experience.

Another was my mother's cousin Asia, the one who came over and massaged me the day after I came home from my banding surgery. Barely five feet tall, she went in at about 190 pounds (Dr. Ren performed the operation) and now is down to 120.

Along with my mother and Asia, there was a friend of Wiggy's—Elizabeth—who was suffering from high blood pressure, respiratory problems, and sore knees. She, too, went for the band after I told her my story—as did Mona, a new receptionist in my doctor's office.

Mona told me once that I was "so beautiful," and when I shared with her how much I used to weigh, she couldn't believe it. She had the surgery only about two months before this writing, but she is already down from the mid two hundreds to the low two hundreds, looking forward to losing much more weight still.

Mona is one of the finest gastric band recipients I've ever come across. She exercises every single day on her lunch break and follows her diet to a tee, to the point that when she went for her first band adjustment six weeks after her surgery, she had already lost twenty-eight pounds.

It's not just people who are one way or another in my circle whom I have influenced to get the band. The first person I didn't know I met at a seminar in Conshohocken, Pennsylvania, a Philly suburb. Drs. Fielding and Ren were there to give a talk at a seminar, and I was there to support the event.

It was about a year after my surgery. I shook many hands that night, but there was one gentleman who came up to me who was really serious. We discussed insurance and other nitty-gritty matters and I even gave him my phone number, telling him that he could call me if he needed help or advice along the way.

About a year later, when I was in the doctors' office for an adjustment, a really thin man came into the waiting room and began staring at me. I noticed he had on a wedding band, so I was offended and turned my head.

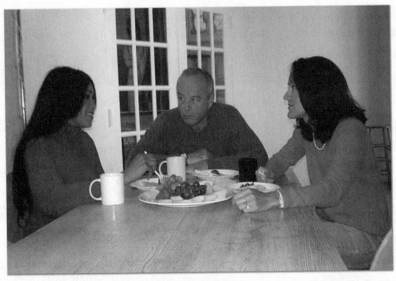

CHATTING WITH DRS. FIELDING AND REN ABOUT GIVING TALKS ON BANDING. WE'RE SNACKING ON—WHAT ELSE?—FRUIT.

He went in for his band fill, then walked over to me as he came back out into the waiting area. I was getting very angry that a married man was hitting on me when he said, "Listen, I just want to thank you."

I didn't know what he was talking about. He then said, "You don't know who I am, do you?"

It was the guy from Conshohocken. He had lost 120 pounds in one year and looked amazing. I simply didn't recognize him.

"You have no idea how my whole life has changed," he told me. "My health is better. My job's better. People treat me better. I never imagined it could be this simple. It has been an amazing year. I threw away my cane, I threw away my medicine. I wanted to tell you how much I appreciate your taking the time with me that night."

I was flabbergasted. But it made me realize I had information that could really help people who had suffered with their weight the way I had.

After that experience, I began to speak more freely to people about my operation. I even gave my cell phone number to some near strangers who brought up the subject of weight or how I looked because I felt it was that important that they contact me if they were sitting on the fence about the band and needed some more information or encouragement. With other problems—gambling, smoking, drinking, and such—people who have managed to put their troubles behind them often feel perfectly free to talk to others in the same boat and try to lend a helping hand. That's true, too, for people who have lost thirty or forty pounds on Weight Watchers. They'll get out there and tell others who want to lose a two-digit number of pounds how they did it. But when it comes to having a surgery to cure obesity, so many people remain mum, as if they went the shameful route. And all that does is keep the stigma attached to it *and* leave those who need to learn about it remaining in the dark.

That's particularly unfortunate in light of the fact that the weight-loss surgery that does get attention in this country—gastric bypass—is more dangerous. It also comes with a greater possibility of at least some weight regain since the stomach stretches after the surgery so the patient eventually feels hungry again and can fit in more food. Carnie Wilson, perhaps the most famous gastric bypass patient, encapsulated the point in the title of a book she wrote a couple of years after her surgery: *I'm Still Hungry*. Well, I'm almost three years out from my surgery, more than 150 pounds lighter than I used to be, and I'm *not* hunrgy.

Don't get me wrong. I applaud Carnie because I know that by going public before many others would, she took on a lot—and has helped countless people. Even with the bypass, most patients don't return to their original weight and are therefore significantly healthier than they used to be. The thing is, the bypass operation *can* begin to fail you after a while.

The band, on the other hand, can't fail you. By going for adjustments whenever you're starting to feel hungry, it never stops working for you. A case in point: Dr. Fielding, by his own admission, had gotten a little sloppy about using his band to keep him trim and had put back some fifteen pounds over time. But seven years after his operation—seven years, mind you—he got serious again, went for his tightenings, and is now walking around in tailored Italian suits with the profile of a fit man in his twenties. The band will always be there for you if you let it.

Another way of putting it: the band is not about hope, as in, "I hope this diet will finally be the one that works." Hope is a killer because it's the opposite of having control over the situation. It's about wishing. Banding, on the other hand, is about results. It *works*. You don't have to hope that it will.

My mother recently gained twenty-seven pounds in a pretty short span of time when she had a break from her band with a total loosening. As she was going to get tightened, she was so upset with herself, lamenting about "having let this happen," and so on. I said, "Mom, relax. You're not *hoping* you'll lose the weight. There's no question that after your fill, you will." I was right. With a band, you "clean up" easy. There are, as I've said before, no more "I blew its."

As for any stigma attached to getting a gastric band, that's crazy. One reason is that there are now more overweight people than healthy-weight people; two in three Americans are carrying around more pounds than is good for them. So who, exactly, is pointing fingers? More important, stigma doesn't help anyone. In fact, it takes the focus away from solutions and keeps obesity intractable by incorrectly casting it as a moral issue (as in "what's wrong with you?"). Even many in the medical community continue to act on the false assumption that obesity is a moral, or willpower, issue, exhorting their very large patients simply to cut calories and exercise more when it's clear that that formula generally fails for knocking off a hundred-plus pounds.

It's not surprising that physicians are often as entrenched in this view as laypeople. Doctors are not divorced from the larger community and can get caught up in the same judgments about willpower and self-control as everyone else.

But morbid obesity is not a character issue; it's a medical one. If Drs. Fielding and Ren were performing surgeries to remove malignancies and eradicate other illnesses that could shorten the life span, no one would question it. On the contrary, the inventor of the gastric band would win the Nobel Prize for medicine since he's responsible for saving hundreds of thousands of lives with bands around the world.

Some people argue that a gastric band isn't really a medical device, like, say, a pacemaker. But isn't it? If you stay morbidly obese, chances are you are going to cut short your life—and, along the way, cost the health care system countless dollars (the dollars *you* spend on your health insurance premiums) in treating every obesity-related condition from diabetes to sleep apnea.

I know it sounds like I'm proselytizing, but I feel I have to argue so fervently precisely because there's so much resistance to this cure. The band has proven such an obvious answer, for so many.

It would be great, of course, if we could get to *prevention* of obesity so that we wouldn't have to get to a cure. But we're not there yet—almost everywhere in the world overweight is surpassing underweight/malnutrition as the most pressing public health problem. Thus, in the meantime, we might as well avail ourselves of the cures available.

I'm not trying to suggest that a gastric band is the only option for someone who is morbidly obese. Everybody has to choose the way that's right for them. The thing is, while there's all this sermonizing and politicking about what very large people should do and what is the right approach by the medical community, there *is* a solution out there that's safe, reasonable, accessible, and, unfortunately, underutilized—in large part because people have decided it's cheating. It's not.

Think about it. No matter what anyone says, your value is not in whether you choose a medical procedure to help you lose weight, so why continue to remain in pain, both physically and emotionally, if you don't have to? Anybody who would say you should because *they've* determined what's a legitimate way for a person to reach her goal is not the sort of person from whom you should be taking your cues in the first place.

10

ON MY WAY

y whole life I dreamed of a fairy-tale ending—being rescued, fitted with a glass slipper as I sat passively. I much
prefer the story the way it actually occurred. I rescued *myself*.

And it wasn't an ending. It was a beginning. When you're overweight, you forever have your life on hold. The most common refrain
running through the mind of a very large person begins, "When I
lose weight . . ." So the tale can't even start. But once you're a healthy
size, and can count on staying that way because of the device inside
you that's going to continually help you control your hunger, you can
begin to determine how your life is going to go. You can start design-
ing the story the way you think it ought to be, and working toward
your dreams.

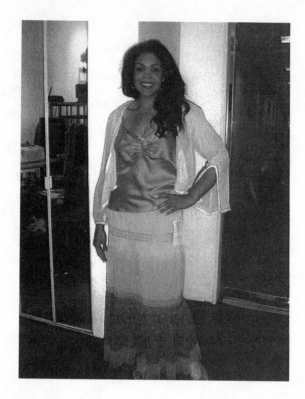

That, I think, is the fairy-tale part of having lost more than 150 pounds. I don't feel stuck anymore. I don't feel like I did at fifteen, when it was difficult to imagine myself in a better future. I feel now that I can create the future I want.

Even without that, there are changes going on all the time that feel great. They're not necessarily huge changes. You don't slay dragons in your fairy-tale-come-true of becoming thin. The dragons just sort of wither by the wayside. Life becomes *normal* in a way it never had been. For instance, when I used to walk onto a crowded elevator, it would bounce up and down a little as I took my place, drawing even more mortifying attention to me than the sight of my heft alone. I used to take great pains to time my steps getting on so I wouldn't create that bobbing motion. Now I can just enter and press the button for my floor without drawing any unflattering attention to myself.

Also, I no longer have to manipulate myself getting in or out of a taxi, a sight people would watch quietly. I can just glide through the open door.

Of course, the drama of those day-to-day changes plays out totally on the inside. It's not like you can tap the shoulder of the person next to you and say, "See, the elevator didn't even shake as I raced in. I'm normal now." But that doesn't make it any less exhilarating.

Admittedly, "normal" is a little different for me. Once people find out you're a daughter of one of the most recognized people on the planet, the whole baseline of whatever is normal changes. But there's "normal" even as Muhammad Ali's child that I wasn't able to enjoy before.

When I would be invited to various red-carpet events, either in my father's honor or simply as a member of the Ali family, people expected something other than a woman who was rotund. Fortunately, because people love my father so much, they refrained from actively hurting me. They would just stare and be quietly polite. And paparazzi never snapped a nasty photo so people could thumb through a magazine and say, "Get a load of . . ." (Of course, my photo didn't make it into any society pages, either.)

Still, it was very hard, since none of my father's other daughters ever struggled with such a severe weight problem. It was particularly hard showing up to events when Laila started boxing. The scrutinizing could get very intense.

Now I don't have to sweat taking my place as my father's daughter. There's not a complicating layer of embarrassment covering public moments. That is a *huge* relief that only someone who has once been fat could understand.

Sometimes it gets even better than "normal." One day when I dropped Jacob off at school I heard a little girl tell her mother, "Jacob's mommy is very pretty. I want to look like her." I held that so close to my heart because children are not good at hiding their shock when a 325-pound woman walks into the room. It used to be very painful for me to see children dropping their jaws when they caught a glimpse of me.

Also, I enjoy noticing men stealing looks. Even women sometimes compliment me, asking if I'm a model. I'm uncomfortable saying it—I know it sounds immodest—but it does happen here and there. And it's so much different from "You have such a pretty face." I used to hear that now and then, and it only served to make me feel bad because the unspoken follow-up to that is, "If only you could lose weight." In other words, "You have such a pretty face" is not really a compliment and not encouraging, either, for someone who wants to slim down. It's just another way of telling a fat girl that she's not acceptable as is.

An even more important difference than the compliments is that I feel less emotionally vulnerable now, less like I have to work extra hard to ward off cruelty because of my size. Part of the stereotype, or perhaps stigma, of being the fat girl is that you're the "nice" one, the one who always says yes—the pleaser, the one who can be counted on. And there definitely still is a part of me who continues to be that girl, the one who doesn't want to disappoint anyone.

But there has been a palpable shift, and I feel the shift continuing still. I don't feel as much as I used to that I somehow have to compensate for being myself by going the extra mile. Don't get me wrong. I truly enjoy doing for others. But it's more for my own sense of the need to do good now and less for someone else's approval. Likewise, I don't feel as much that I have to fill voids when there's silence or feel worried and try to "fix" things if I said something that someone else may not have agreed with.

I have to say, this is one of the most freeing aspects of my weight loss, even more freeing than not having to make my way through life gasping for breath and having to sit down to rest all the time. Constantly feeling like I was the one who had to make everyone else happy was *exhausting,* much more exhausting, in fact, than carrying around the extra weight could ever be. It left me no mental energy for myself. I had no reserve to tend to my projects at full throttle.

It's ironic to me to feel stronger as a smaller person, to feel less like I'm going to get hurt. I have armor now—good, sustaining armor—that all those layers of fat were not able to provide.

More ironic still, my newfound strength has made me more open to receiving. Before, I had a hard time accepting anything from anyone, whether a compliment, a gift, or a favor. I guess I was afraid the balance in a relationship would be shifted away from me if I was given to, like I wouldn't have any leverage. Now I see relationships less as about having leverage, about protecting myself, and more about the healthy give-and-take they should be.

I don't mean to imply with the changes I've been experiencing that everything in my life is now perfect because I've arrived at a healthy weight. There are still times, for instance, when I want to eat for emotional reasons, or crave a food that is high in calories or that doesn't work well with the band. But it's much easier now to ride out the wave of a craving without giving in. It has become more of a *pattern* for me now, a *habit,* to purposefully engage in something other than eating when an impulse to eat pops up. I make a phone call, or tend to some paperwork, or get up from where I'm sitting and take a short walk, even as short as five minutes. My solutions may sound simple, but they work extremely well because they're incompatible with putting food in your mouth. And I can overcome food cravings with ease using these distractions because I have proven to myself so many times now that they really do work. Just a few minutes away from a desire to eat loosens the desire's hold, as long as you're not truly hungry.

Other aspects of my life that I'm less satisfied about, and haven't yet hit upon solutions to, include various parts of my body. One of them is my skin, and I very much want to get skin surgery.

My skin isn't as much of an issue as it tends to be for people who have lost three hundred or four hundred pounds. In those cases, the apron of skin hanging over the stomach can be so big it hangs below the genitals. Like a rubber band that has been stretched for too long, it just doesn't snap back, and people who have lost hundreds of pounds literally have to fold their skin flap into their skirt or pants. The extra skin (think of shar-peis, those wrinkly-looking dogs) also makes such people prone to rashes, fungal infections, chafing, sores, even back pain in some cases.

Still, while my situation isn't as severe, I do have rolls of loose skin over my middle—a sack—that I can grab in my hands, and I have the same type of skin sagging under my arms. It's sort of crepe paper–like. There's even a little excess skin hanging on certain parts of my legs. It simply hasn't shrunk as well as the rest of me.

My breasts now sag, too—they breast-fed, went up to an E cup in my mid-twenties, and then down to what is now a C cup—so they lost a good deal of their elasticity. And at thirty-two years old, I'm not willing to say, "Oh well, they sag, but that's okay." I'm too young for them to have gone south permanently. I want implants to help support them, to achieve what breasts should look like in a woman my age.

People have said to me that my desire for skin and breast surgery is frivolous. Some have even asked me point-blank if I've developed an eating disorder since I lost the weight in some kind of quest for perfection. They think that because you're not 100 percent satisfied with the dramatic changes to your body after the gastric band, you must have some kind of mental problem.

It's incredibly unfair. I have a right to want to go sleeveless, which I can't do now because of the skin sagging on my arms. I have a right to feel comfortable with my nudity instead of always having to deal with the excess weight I once had because of the flap of skin on my stomach. I have a right to like the body I look at.

And skin surgery is no walk in the park, so it's not like I haven't done a lot of thinking about this. For one thing, there's the expense. It can cost upward of $65,000, even $100,000 in some cases, and insurance rarely covers it. You have to document how you have suffered from excess skin for at least a year, keeping notes on skin diseases and rashes. And even *then*, many people are declined.

If you do go through with the surgery—covered by insurance or not—it often doesn't happen in one bout. The procedures take place gradually over time, maybe starting with the stomach, lower back, and buttocks in one session and then going back for more cutting and anesthesia to take care of the breasts and arms. In some cases, there could be a third surgery to cut away skin from the inner thighs. And recovery can be painful and consist of weeks of swelling and time off from your routine.

In addition, many people who undergo skin surgery end up with long, noticeable scars for life around the back and abdomen (you can look like you were cut in half and sewn back together) or up and down the limbs. In other words, you can't completely erase your past, particularly when you want to get intimate with someone.

Nevertheless, the skin is the largest organ on the body—yes, it's an organ—and I deserve to get my excess eight to ten pounds of it cut off, despite the flak I've gotten for wanting to take care of it. For me, it's an essential part of the journey. So I continue to talk to different plastic surgeons about skin surgery and read up about its aftermath. I know it's another chapter I will be writing for myself.

At the same time that I'm dissatisfied with how my skin looks, I haven't completely caught up to my thinner self—the part of my banding surgery that I'm thrilled about. Yes, when I look in the mirror, I see a strong, healthy woman, but a part of me still feels fat. Psychologists who study people who have undergone weight-loss surgery would say I'm typical, that it takes a while for your mind to catch up with your new, smaller size and that some people even need sessions with a therapist to adjust. I guess even now, almost three years out, I still have some catching up to do.

Another thing I have to adjust to with the weight loss, aside from the weight loss itself, is that I sometimes sense a cattiness from other women that didn't used to be. I suppose that when you're obese, you're in no way seen as social competition, but once you're in the game, there can be a coldness that I hadn't experienced.

I'm no longer a part of the fat pack, either, and since that was even my role professionally, it takes some getting used to. There's a whole subculture of very overweight women who support one another, and I don't have that now. In fact, at shows for my plus-size clothing patterns, large women have even come up to me and berated me for having lost the weight, as if I've sold out on them. It's difficult, because I haven't sold out. I've done what's right for *me,* as I've explained over and over.

A lot of large women, I think, have given me a hard time out of defensiveness, so they have some catching up with themselves to do. But women who truly don't want to work on losing weight shouldn't. I've never tried to change anyone's mind. I hold myself up only as an example of someone who always wanted a solution to excess weight but hadn't been able to find an acceptable one before learning about the band.

Also on the adjusting-to-healthy-weight agenda is my not yet having found a man I want to share my life with. I'd be lying if I said I wasn't hoping that there's a Prince Charming out there for me. There's a part of every woman, I think, that wants to be swept off her feet. But my prince would need to accept me being self-sufficient—I want to be swept, not rescued.

Also, he'd need to want a wife, not a father-in-law. So many men I've met have wanted to get close to me simply because of who my father is—or, on the flip side, have been intimidated because of who he is. At this point, I will accept into my life only someone with whom *I* share an intimate connection, not someone who feels the connection is either enhanced or complicated by my father's renown.

I suppose that in the back of my mind I thought losing the excess weight would somehow make finding a soul mate easier. It has made *dating* easier, more by boosting my confidence than anything else. But soul mate—that's a whole different thing.

The wait is okay, though. I'd like it—someone to come home to at the end of the day—but I'm not preoccupied with it. Romance is only one aspect of a very full life, and it will come when it comes. It's not an issue you can force.

In the meantime, I'm enjoying all the good parts of the very full life I am living. In particular, I've been thrilled with how my charity work has been going—and by the good feedback I've been receiving. Last May 25, National Missing Children's Day, I was presented by the United States attorney general with the Volunteer of the Year award, which is bestowed by the Department of Justice to someone for efforts on behalf of those boys and girls who have been abducted. More than two thousand children are reported missing every single day, and the work of the National Center for Missing and Exploited Children, to which I lend my services, has resulted in the recovery of more than eighty-seven thousand of them.

I was also lucky enough, through my charity work, to finally get to meet Dionne Warwick. For some time now I have been involved with a New York–based organization called Project Sunshine, which provides free programs and services to children (and their families) with cancer, AIDS, and other serious medical challenges. One thing

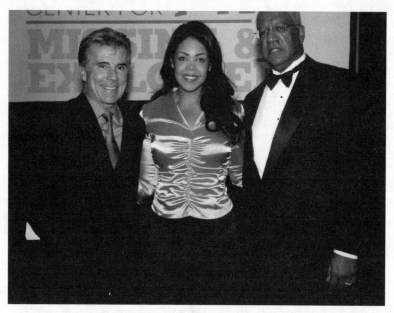

AT AN EVENT FOR THE NATIONAL CENTER FOR MISSING AND EXPLOITED CHILDREN.
JOHN WALSH, ON THE LEFT, IS ONE OF THE FOUNDERS, AND HERBERT C.
JONES, ON THE RIGHT, IS VICE PRESIDENT OF EXTERNAL AFFAIRS.
Courtesy National Center for Missing and Exploited Children.

I have been able to do for them is get people in the sports world to donate trophies and such for Project Sunshine's auctions, the proceeds of which go to fund various programs to help families through devastating health crises.

Well, Dionne Warwick happens to be on Project Sunshine's board of directors, and last May, at a benefit dinner at the Waldorf-Astoria, Project Sunshine founder Joe Weilgus made sure we were introduced. He knew how much I admire her and how much I love her music and went out of his way to ensure a face-to-face meeting.

The icing on the cake was that she sang at the event! There I was, two tables away, as she performed "That's What Friends Are For," and of course I started crying as soon as I heard the first strains. Then Joe grabbed me and a few other people onto the stage as she started sing-

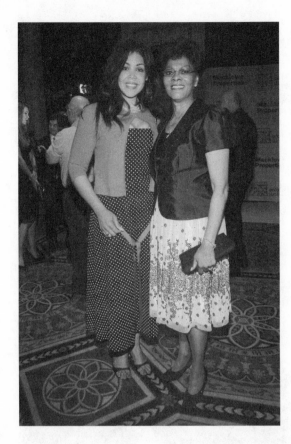

ing "What the World Needs Now." We all just hugged and sang along with her, me still crying and also holding Jacob and my sister Jenna, who were with me that night.

Even better was that I got to tell her how much she meant to me, how much her music always helped me when I needed something beautiful to hold on to. She hugged and kissed me and told me it was so good to see me and asked how I was. I was amazed that she remembered me. And she said "what a beautiful, beautiful boy" Jacob was, which only added to the wonderful emotions.

Along with the good things that are coming from my charity work, I'm aiming to get a new clothing line off the ground. The Simplicity sewing patterns continue to be popular, not just in plus sizes but for smaller women, too. But I'd also like to have a label of my own, and continue to speak to various designers about it. My aim is to devote 10 percent of my earnings to various charities, which would bring my love of fashion full circle with the unspoken mandate my father has given to me to help others.

In the meantime, I continue to take each day as it comes, even while I work to pull various projects together. I enjoy raising my son, who's now in the second grade, and seeing my friends and family. I enjoy working out, which I can do in a way I never even used to be able to dream of. I enjoy meeting people and making friends through my charity work and my work on the Simplicity line.

What runs through all of it, heightening the good feelings, is the knowledge that I will never again have to worry about being overweight. The band will always protect me, so I don't have to be at war

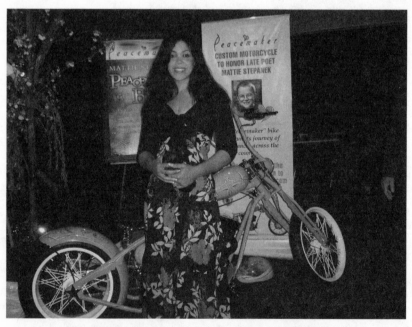

THE "PEACEMAKER" BIKE BEHIND ME IS USED TO RAISE AWARENESS FOR THE MUSCULAR DYSTROPHY ASSOCIATION'S MATTIE FUND. Courtesy LynnJonesFoundation.org

with my body anymore. It also makes me feel *confident*. When you're fat, that's all you are. It's what people see first and how they label you, even after you prove yourself to them. At a healthy weight, the "fat" label disappears and no longer takes over people's impressions of you.

The band makes me feel *calm,* too—at ease. Before, there was always the disturbing hum of my weight in the background. I couldn't take pleasure in any of life's joys without experiencing creeping anxiety from the thought "This would be so much better if only . . ." Now I can delight in the good things with serenity. By the same token, I can meet life's challenges more productively because my energy is not being spent on my weight. What I mean is, without the excess baggage of weight, both emotional and physical, the highs are even higher because there's nothing to drag them down, and the lows are blunted because they're not complicated by an ever-present handicap.

It's not, as Sri Chinmoy wished for me, that all my dreams have come true. I don't think you ever cross a finish line in that way. But I can create opportunities for myself that I wouldn't have been able to before, working productively toward them. I can be *susceptible* to happiness, to achieving my goals. I can allow myself to feel *blessed,* more ready than ever to reach out to others; *eligible,* ready to be reached out to; and *worthy,* secure in my own value.

Good things are coming, I know it. They are for you, too.

ACKNOWLEDGMENTS

Everyone who worked on this book would like to thank Peggy Tagliarino of Peggy Tagliarino Public Relations, who was lining up the eight ball to go in the corner pocket before any of us had even picked up our cue sticks. Many thanks, too, to our agent, Wendy Weil, who believed in this project from the get-go and worked her magic to make all the elements fall into place. And to our editor at HarperCollins, Mary Ellen O'Neill, our appreciation for letting us convince her that what we had to say needed to get heard.

Khaliah thanks: God, because I don't believe any of this just happened; Spencer Wertheimer, for giving me my son, and for everything else, which I could never even attempt to articulate; my mother, who is both mother and best friend, in all the good guises and bad, and I cherish the whole lot of it; my grandmother Dorothy, for the love, the support, the grape soda—I hope you know you are more mother than grandmother to me and that so many of the ways I'm grounded I owe to you; my siblings Jared, Jenna, and Lydia, for everything we have shared and will continue to share, all of it filled with my love for you; and Joe Abrams, my brother—it doesn't matter that we don't share parents—who has nourished me and saved me more times and in more types of situations than I could ever count. I also thank my "brother" Jonny Abrams, whose support transcends description, and Jennifer and Ethel Abrams for all the good light they shed. My siblings Maryum, Rasheeda, Jamilla, Muhammad Jr., Miya, Hana, Laila, and Asaad, you are the bright stars in whose reflection I glow. Cousin Ivana, you are my copilot. Thanks for always sitting with me in the cockpit and never bailing out. Uncle Kelly, thanks for bringing me into this world and for always being there as I make my way through it. Aunt Rose and Little Teddy, you two are closer than blood to me. Uncle Luqman, what you have given me has kept me going more times than you could ever realize. Larry Fletcher, my stepfather, my love to you for stepping in. Mary Duffy, if you hadn't bothered to take notice, I don't know what would have happened. Ditto to Bill Ford—thank you for believing in me and standing by me. George and Christine, my surgeons, thank God I found you. You helped me attain not only the body I wasn't able to attain on my own but also your friendship—who could have anticipated? Gaspar Rosario, Gio Dugay, Mary Occean, Beth Abrams, Priscilla Cintron, and Dr. Fredericks, you are the glue that has held everything together. Larry Lindner, your ability to channel my thoughts and feelings and bring them to paper amazes me. Thanks, friend, for all the midnight powwows after your son and mine were finally asleep. I love you. Joe Weilgus, I can't even begin to express appreciation for your always going above and beyond, not just for me but also for my son. Bonnie Simmons and Judy Raymond of Simplicity, have I thanked you enough? Is it possible to thank you enough? Kenneth Cole, Maria Cuomo Cole, do I really know you two? It's too amazing for words. Donnis Honeycutt, your warmth and guidance mean so much. Jacqui Frazier-Lyde, my dear friend and sister, thanks for proving with me that good feelings run deeper than enmity. Wiggy Olson, gratitude to you for pointing me in the right direction when I felt there was no direction left to choose. Lou Schwartz and Stan Smith, without your opening the gates in New York, it wouldn't have all gotten started. Sri Chinmoy, for the way you have calmed me and lifted me at the same time, I'll always be grateful. Dr. Reverend Schuller, for almost two decades you have been supporting and strengthening me through your program. Alan Buchman, you have opened so many avenues. Sunjay Rawls, your help has been invaluable. Rafi Nasser and Robert and Dongmei Peng, gratitude for the spiritual lifting. Robin Moran, thanks for the love. Dr. Meilahn, it means more than you know that you take care of me. Dr. Stephen Soloway and family, you are such wonderful friends. I love you all. Vernon Vincent, I am honored to know you and indebted for your helping to educate people about the gastric band. Ismail Numan, my amazing trainer, thanks for picking up where the band leaves off. Mina Williford, my guardian angel, my deepest appreciation for loving me and looking after me when I was in need. Grandmom Vivian, Great-Grandmom Reba, Grandmom Odessa, Grandmom Rose, Camille Ewald, and Brian and Darnell Parker, you can't talk to me anymore, but I talk to you and draw strength from you every single day. Thank you, as always. Naomi Ramsey, gratitude for your always being in my corner. Finally, Dad, thanks for the legacy, which I hope to live up to. It's a blessing and honor to be your child.

Dr. George Fielding thanks: Vern Vincent, for inventing the Lap-Band, and for his unstinting efforts in educating surgeons around the world; Professor Paul O'Brien, for introducing me to the band and for doing mine; my friends and colleagues in Brisbane; Dr. Jennifer Duncombe, for looking after my Brisbane patients; my children, Stephanie, Andrew, James, and Samantha, who mean more to me than words could express; and my wife, Christine Ren, with whom every day is a new beginning that I eagerly look forward to.

Dr. Christine Ren thanks: my mentor, H. Leon Pachter, without whom I wouldn't have this public forum to acknowledge him; my office staff, aka the world's best team players; my parents, Sam and Lucy Ren, who gave me everything I needed to become the person I wanted to be; and my husband, George Fielding, who is there for me in a way that I used to think happened only in storybooks.

Larry Lindner thanks: Khaliah, who honored me with her trust enough to share her life with me, no matter how painful or private; and who has taught me so much, including that celebrity, viewed up close, is a lot different from what it looks like glimpsed from the crowd. I love you, too. Thanks, too, to Drs. Fielding and Ren, who perform top-notch surgery like, well, like top-notch surgeons, but who translate complicated medical information like talk-show hosts. To my son, John, gratitude for filling my heart in ways you won't possibly be able to understand until you become a parent yourself; and love and everything else to my wife, Constance, without whom, what would be the point?

I have been involved with more than two dozen charities over the years. Here are some of the ones whose missions I've worked on particularly closely or felt particularly keenly about. They don't just need money; they need your time.

National Center for Missing and Exploited Children
Charles B. Wang International Children's Building
699 Prince Street
Alexandria, VA 22314-3175
703-274-3900
www.missingkids.com
    Our children are our most valuable resource. When even one is missing, it's a crisis, but more than two thousand children are reported missing *every single day*. This organization works in cooperation with the Department of Justice to find them, provide services for families, and also to prevent child sexual exploitation.

HELP USA
5 Hanover Square, 17th floor

New York, NY 10004

800-311-7999

www.helpusa.org

HELP USA empowers homeless people and others in need to become and remain self-sufficient. In addition to providing quality housing, this organization provides on-site support services, including employment training, life skills education, child care, substance abuse counseling, and much, much more.

Project Sunshine

102 West 38th Street, 8th floor

New York, NY 10018

212-354-8035

www.projectsunshine.org

Project Sunshine provides free programs and services to children affected with such illnesses as cancer, AIDS, and other serious medical challenges. College students, artists, lawyers, executives, actors, and people from all kinds of other backgrounds donate their time to improve the lives of the children (and their families) Project Sunshine serves.

We Are Family Foundation

320 West 37th Street, 8th floor

New York, NY 10018

212-397-4333

www.wearefamilyfoundation.org

In a world where conflict and misunderstanding between cultures, religious groups, and countries dominate the landscape, the We Are Family Foundation provides a message of hope by promoting our common humanity through early-childhood-education initiatives and various media resources. There are now twelve We are Family schools and six student treks. Giving of yourself to this worthy organization is a great way to foster mutual respect and appreciation of cultural diversity.

Culture Project
55 Mercer Street
New York, NY 10013
212-253-7017
www.cultureproject.com

This unique organization gives voice to the marginalized in our society by staging plays that dramatize their plight. For instance, it put on a play called *The Exonerated* that focused attention on six wrongfully imprisoned exonerees, who were finally released (in some cases, after decades) without recognition of wrongdoing or compensation. The play, produced in New York, was made into a movie with Brian Dennehy, Susan Sarandon, Danny Glover, and Aidan Quinn.

Culture Project productions, performed at 55 Mercer Street, have won the Freedom of Expression Award from Amnesty International and the PASS award from the National Association of Criminal Defenders.

Soup's On!
4050 Conshohocken Avenue
Philadelphia, PA 19131
215-452-0430

Run by my dear friend Wiggy (Arlene) Olson, Soup's On! is the only self-supporting project of the Salvation Army. The program trains people who have ended up down-and-out for careers in catering and other food service positions. The job retention rate for "graduates" of Soup's On! is 94 percent, and men and women who were once on drugs or in other hard-knocks situations end up catering events for such outfits as the Philadelphia Opera Company.

Big Brothers Big Sisters of America
230 North 13th Street
Philadelphia, PA 19107
215-567-7000
www.bbbs.org

Children mentored by a volunteer big brother or sister are 46 percent less likely to begin using illegal drugs and 52 percent less likely to skip school. Being a big sibling is not overwhelming. It takes only a few hours a month of hanging out and talking, walking together in the park, sharing a pizza, or playing a board game or some ball. The organization matches each volunteer with a child six to eighteen in a professionally supported one-to-one relationship.

Communities in Schools
277 South Washington Street, Suite 210
Alexandria, VA 22314
800-CIS-4KIDS
www.cisnet.org

Every child needs the resources that make the difference between a graduate and a dropout. Communities in Schools provides them. This organization helps kids stay in school with the "Five Basics": a personal relationship with a caring adult, perhaps via a mentor or parental involvement program; a safe place, such as an after-school or extended-hours program; a healthy start that might include anything from mental health counseling to family strengthening initiatives to dental exams; a marketable skill, provided in the form of technology training, career counseling or college preparation; and a chance to give back through community service opportunities and other venues.

National Association of Police Athletics/Activities Leagues (PAL) Inc.
658 West Indiantown Road, Suite #201
Jupiter, FL 33458

561-745-5535
www.nationalpal.org

PAL helps prevent juvenile crime and violence by providing civic, athletic, recreational, and educational resources for children. In so doing, this organization creates trust and understanding between police officers and youths, improving communities as it improves lives. In other words, kids who grow up with PAL learn responsible values and attitudes, which leads to good citizenship.

Lupus Foundation of America, Inc.
2000 L Street, NW, Suite 710
Washington, DC 20036
202-349-1155
www.lupus.org

My mother is one of an estimated 1.5 million Americans who suffer with lupus, a chronic inflammatory disease that can affect various parts of the body, especially the skin, joints, blood, and kidneys. It is ten to fifteen times more common in women than in men. The Lupus Foundation is dedicated to finding both cause(s) and cure.

Wildlife Warriors Worldwide
P.O. Box 29
Beerwah QLD 4519
Australia
61 7 5436 2026
www.wildlifewarriors.org

Initially established in 2002 by Steve Irwin and his wife, Terri, Wildlife Warriors supports the protection of injured, threatened, or endangered wildlife. It also works to protect the natural environment and undertakes biological research, among other animal-saving initiatives.

obesity surgery (*continued*)
   See also gastric banding references;
     Khaliah's surgery references
Olson, Arlene "Wiggy," 79–80, 142

Patient Financial Services, 104
patient follow-up, 4
Patinkin, Mandy, 138
Pauley, Jane, 7, 28–29, 36, 65, 140
payment options, 101–4
   alternative help, 104
   insurance, 101–4
Pendergrass, "Mama Rose," 15, 27
Pendergrass, Teddy, Jr., 16–17, 24
People Are Talking appearance, 28
People for the American Way
   appearance, 137–38
perfume business, 44
period, affecting hunger levels,
   146–47, 174
photographs
   avoiding/resenting being in, 56, 72,
    78
   comfort in having taken, 150–51
Pitt, Brad, 153
political campaigning, 55
postoperative problem rate, 4
postoperative protocol. *See* gastric
   banding (recovery)
pregnancy
   with gastric band, 108, 124, 125
   of Khaliah, traumatic experiences,
    67
   safety, gastric banding and, 5
pre-op protocol, 99–100. *See also*
   gastric banding (candidacy and
   pre-op)
problem solving, improved abilities,
   143
Project Sunshine, 209–10, 220
psychologist evaluation, 92, 105
public service award ceremony (with
   Sri Chinmoy), 93–95

questions
   to ask prospective surgeons, 97–99
   frequently asked, about gastric
    banding, 107–9

race
   derogatory comments on, 26, 27,
    37, 56
   mixed background, 24
   only child of color in school, 36–37
   outside perceptions of Khaliah,
    24–25
race, obesity and, 181–91
   comparative figures, 183
   increased health problems and,
    186–87
   universal two-hundred-pound
    milestone, 189
   See also African Americans
Rappin', hosting, 53
Rasheeda (sister), 151
Reba (great-grandmother), 20, 67
recovery time, 5–6
Ren, Dr. Christine
   Khaliah meeting, 2–3, 89
   perspective on surgery, 6
   photograph, 195
respect
   obese people not getting, 10–11, 13,
    182
   reclaiming, 12
responsibility, for weight control
   gastric banding and, 96
   refusing, fueling hunger (physical
    and spiritual), 76
   shirking, victim mentality and, 76
   taking, 11–12
reversibility, of gastric banding, 3, 127
Rosario, Gaspar, 114, 115
Rosemont College, 55–56
Roux-En Y. *See* gastric bypass
Rowe, Jacqueline, 132
ruby ring, receiving, 54

Khaliah Ali, daughter of Muhammad Ali, is an Emmy-nominated talk-show host. A former Ford model, she also has a line of sewing patterns at Simplicity Pattern Company (www.simplicity.com). Her charity work includes serving as chair of the National Center for Missing and Exploited Children's "Hand in Hand with Children" campaign, for which she won the Volunteer of the Year award from the U.S. Department of Justice. In addition, she serves on the board of directors of Help USA and as a spokesperson for Soup's On!, a Salvation Army initiative, along with serving as national spokesperson for Communities in Schools, and participates in many other charitable causes and mentoring programs. She lives with her son in the Philadelphia area.

Dr. George Fielding is one of the world's foremost laparoscopic surgeons. An associate professor in the Department of Surgery at the NYU Medical Center as well as one of the heads of the NYU Program for Surgical Weight Loss, he trained in Australia, Britain, and Switzerland and has taken an active role in teaching laparoscopic surgery to physicians in the United States, Japan, and various other Asian and European countries. He has performed more than four thousand gastric band surgeries, including on the super-obese, and also is the world's most experienced surgeon operating on obese children.

Dr. Fielding is a fellow of the Royal Australasian College of Surgeons and Britain's Royal College of Surgeons. Along with having published more than 150 journal articles, abstracts, and book chapters, he has appeared in numerous venues for the lay public, both in print and electronic media. These include the *Today* show, *The Jane Pauley Show, 60 Minutes Australia,* the *New York Times,* the *New York Post, Newsday,* the *Weekend Australian* magazine, and *Who* magazine. He lives with his wife in New York City.

Dr. Christine Ren is the leading gastric band surgeon in the United States next to Dr. Fielding. Director of the NYU Program for Surgical Weight Loss as well as an assistant professor at NYU Medical Center, Dr. Ren has presented her research on laparoscopic bariatric surgery both nationally and internationally. She is also the chair of the Insurance Committee for the American Society for Bariatric Surgery, the premier organization for bariatric surgeons in the United States.

Dr. Ren has been recognized as one of New York's premier female surgeons by being awarded the YWCA Woman's Achievement Award in 2003 and by being named one of the top forty achievers in New York City under forty years of age by *Crane's New York Business* magazine. She has appeared on *Oprah, Dateline, CBS-TV, Good Day New York,* and in a variety of magazines and newspapers, including *Vogue, Shape, Good Housekeeping, Allure, New York* magazine, and the New York *Daily News.* She lives with her husband in New York City.

Lawrence Lindner is a *New York Times* best-selling coauthor and collaborating writer on a wide variety of books on health and other topics. In addition, Lindner penned a nationally syndicated biweekly column in the the *Washington Post* for several years and wrote a monthly column for the *Boston Globe* from 2004 to 2005. His freelance work has appeared in many publications, including *Condé Nast Traveler, The International Herald Tribune, Woman's Day, McCall's, Eating Well, The New York Post, The Seattle Times, and Reader's Digest*. He lives with his wife and son in Hingham, Massachusetts.